Dr. Bob Arnot's Guide
to Turning Back the Clock

Also by Robert Arnot, M.D.

THE BEST MEDICINE

with Charles Gaines

SPORTSELECTION

SPORTSTALENT

Dr. Bob Arnot's Guide to Turning Back the Clock

ROBERT ARNOT, M.D.

LITTLE, BROWN AND COMPANY
Boston New York Toronto London

First Paperback Edition

Consult your personal physician before beginning any diet and exercise program.

Glycemic Index Table from "Timing and method of increased carbohydrate intake to cope with heavy training, competition and recovery" by E. F. Coyle in the *Journal of Sports Sciences* 1991; 9/spec no: 29–51; reprinted by permission. "Best Vegetables" and "Healthiest Vegetables" December 1991. "Best Fruits" May 1992. "Best Grains" April 1993. "Best Beans" May 1993. "Chinese Report" September 1993. "Italian Report" January/February 1994. From the *Nutrition Action Healthletter.* Copyright © by Center for Science in the Public Interest. Reprinted by permission of CSPI (1875 Connecticut Ave., N.W., Suite 300, Washington, DC 10009-5728. $24.00 for 10 issues).

Library of Congress Cataloging-in-Publication Data
Arnot, Robert Burns.
    Dr. Bob Arnot's guide to turning back the clock / Robert Arnot.—
1st ed.
      p.   cm.
    ISBN 0-316-05189-6 (hc) 0-316-05174-8 (pb)
    1. Middle-aged men—Health and hygiene. 2. Physical fitness for
men. 3. Longevity. 4. Middle-aged men—Nutrition.   I. Title.
RA777.8.A76 1995
613'.04234—dc20   94-40644

10 9 8 7 6 5 4 3 2 1

MV-NY

Published simultaneously in Canada by Little, Brown & Company (Canada) Limited

Printed in the United States of America

To my parents,
who through their vigor and enthusiasm have shown our
family how to remain young and strong through old age.
To my children, Bobby and Hayden,
who every day motivate my wife, Courtney, and me
to do the same.

Contents

CONTENTS

Acknowledgments

I would like to thank Jill Werman, whose skillful insight, dedication, and perseverance made this book possible. Her know-how and intelligence provided the cutting-edge research that has added so much value to this book. I am truly grateful for her partnership.

Thanks also to my editor at Little Brown, Jennifer Josephy, and her assistant, Abigail Wilentz, for their tireless efforts, enthusiasm, and cheerfulness.

And to my agents Dan and Simon Green for making this book happen.

The experts I interviewed for this book were extremely gracious with their time and knowledge. I would like to offer special thanks to the following people for extending themselves on so many occasions: Clayton Abrams, Steve Blechman, Richard Bothwell, Vic Braden, Bread & Circus Whole Foods Market, Dr. Luke Bucci, the Center for Science in the Public Interest, Dr. Michael Colgan, Dr. Ed Coyle, Dr. Chuck Dillman, John Douglas, Dr. Bill Evans, Gary Fisher, Charles Gaines, Ben Gaylord, Juliann Goldman, Rick Grogan, Andrew Hall, Lee Haney, Austin Hearst, Dr. Charles H. Hennekens, Ed Irace, C.P.T., Dr. John Ivy, Gary Kiedaisch, John Kukoda, Bob LeMond, Tony Marabella, Dave Merriam, the Mount Mansfield Ski

Resort and Cross Country Ski Center, Nick Bollettieri Tennis Academy, Jon Niednagel, Eric Ober, Oldways Preservation & Exchange Trust, Ned Overend, Michael Radutzky, the Royal Gorge Cross Country Ski Resort, Arnold Schwarzenegger, Jeanne Soper, Toga Bike Shop, the Trapp Family Lodge Cross Country Ski Center, Vail Ski School, Jim Vandergrift, Rob Vandermark, the Vic Braden Tennis College, Jim and Phil Wharton, Dr. Keith Wheeler, Warren Witherell, World Gym at Lincoln Center, and my daily cycle-training partner, Bobby Arnot.

THE GAME PLAN

Chapter 1

Turning Back the Clock

IN 1987, I FLEW TO SAN FRANCISCO FOR A DAY OF TRAINING WITH America's oldest living teenager, octogenarian Walt Stack, a man whose fame derives less from what he does than how he does it.

Walt met our CBS camera crew at the Dolphin Swim Club after completing his 2:00 A.M. fifty-mile morning bike ride. I joined Walt for his seventeen-mile daily training run over the Golden Gate Bridge, down through Sausalito, and then back to the Dolphin Club. Next event, a swim in the 54-degree waters of San Francisco harbor, across from Alcatraz, where he was once a guest of the federal government. Walt jumped in with no more than a rumpled swimsuit and a white swim cap. He swam over a mile in forty-five minutes. I donned a three-quarter-inch neoprene wetsuit complete with hood, booties, and gloves and swam the fastest nine seconds of my life. This wasn't the first time Walt had put a far younger man to shame. One week, building toward his one-hundred-marathon personal record, he completed the 26.2-mile Boston event, flew through the night on a red-eye, and raced again at 8:00 A.M. in California. At the twenty-four-mile mark of that Santa Rosa event, Walt punished a competitor half his age, who had tried to pass him, by tossing a can of beer over his shoulder, remarking "guess that finishes the six-pack," and accelerating away from him.

After our swim, I took Walt to an exercise physiology laboratory. I asked the doctor in charge to run a maximum-oxygen-consumption test on Walt, an excellent measure of biological age. The test showed that Walt was an extraordinarily fit and healthy fifty-eight-year-old! That's twenty-six years younger than his birth certificate would lead you to believe. Walt wasn't alone. Thousands of men have cranked their biological clocks back by decades. Others have held their biological age in their early twenties as their birth-certified age crept into their fifties.

Conventional Wisdom:
Go with the flow.
New Paradigm:
Aging is a cultural trap that programs men to abuse, misuse, and disuse their bodies.

How many times have you wished to be eighteen again, taking back with you your wisdom, experience, knowledge, and your wallet? That trip back in time was science fiction a generation ago. Today, returning to your youth can be a reality. If you are between thirty and sixty, you can crank back the time on your biological clock by a staggering amount as determined by standardized human-performance tests for biological age. Between sixty and ninety big gains can still be made. What's changed? Dramatic breakthroughs in nutrition, fitness technology, and sports medicine. If the idea of dragging your body back through a time warp seems like a pretty weird idea, be assured, it really works.

The twenties are your last decade of maintenance-free living. You can drink, party, stay out all night, eat trash foods, yet still pick up a sport at a moment's notice and show dazzling athletic prowess with little conditioning. But beginning in your thirties, body bits and pieces begin to fall apart. Your recovery slows after a hard Saturday and Sunday as a weekend warrior. You can't sprint as fast. Beginning at forty, the sedentary male will lose six pounds of muscle, nearly 7 percent of heart function, and 8 percent of lung function every ten years. Many men accept those events as an inevitable genetically programmed disintegration. Misuse and abuse are widely misinterpreted as aging. The same misfortune would befall a poorly maintained car. After 30,000 maintenance-free miles, many cars will begin to deteriorate if they are not properly cared for. Yet that same car may go to 150,000 miles if meticulously maintained.

I call the twenties the gold standard, since they represent the decade during which we functioned best. Rather than setting shallow fitness goals, resolve to function as if you were still in your twenties. When I enter mountain biking, skiing, cycling, or speed-skating races, I race in the eighteen to thirty group, although I'm forty-seven. I want to be biologically twenty-five. Competing with and beating kids that age is proof of the pudding.

You can set back your biological age, like rolling back the miles on a car's odometer. How much? A sedentary forty- or fifty-year-old can realistically expect to test as a sedentary twenty-five-year-old after as little as six months. How long can you keep your biological age young? A. B. Dill, founder of the Harvard Fatigue Lab, tested himself every year for thirty years and never saw any change in his biological age, as measured by a standard oxygen-consumption test. Dr. Dave Costill, head of the Human Performance Lab at Ball State University, found that runners in their fifties showed little decrease in their performance on standardized tests when compared to their twenties. So it is possible to maintain the performance of a twenty-year-old in your early fifties! "If they're willing to train with the same intensity and volume as the twenty-year-old, we find very little decay in any of their physiology," says Dr. Costill. George Sheehan, the famous running doctor, ran his best marathon ever at age sixty, covering the 26.2-mile course in nearly three hours flat. Age thirty used to be the dreaded end of an athlete's career. Now it's the halfway mark.

Can everyone expect to reset his clock? No. Men who are in seriously good shape and already biologically in their twenties can't expect to budge their clocks more than a couple of years. The men who will undergo the greatest changes are the following:

- Any man who doesn't practice optimum nutrition.
- Sedentary men.
- Aerobically fit men who have never built any muscle.
- Muscularly fit men who are aerobically unfit.

Even men who have physical disabilities that prevent them from using their lower extremities can expect large gains by developing their upper bodies, since most of the body's muscle is above the waist. Charles Gaines, author of *Pumping Iron,* developed enormous aerobic power in his upper body while recovering from a dual hip replacement.

THE TWIN ENGINES OF YOUTH

I fly a twin-engine propeller airplane. With both engines operating, the plane has spectacular performance. It can climb to 25,000 feet and cruise at nearly 300 mph. I've twice lost an engine in flight and have learned that it can fly on the one good engine, but its performance is drastically reduced. Even though the good engine performs extremely well, the plane limps along barely able to climb. The airspeed drops to a crawl. If you choose to develop aerobic fitness as your main engine of youth, you will limp along toward old age. If you choose only to weight train, you'll do better than limp, but not much. Youth requires that you develop those twin engines of fitness.

Top researchers on aging define the twin engines of youth as a large oxygen transport system and a large, lean muscle mass. Both are highly accurate measures of your biological age based on widely accepted scientific tests. Researchers in Boston at the USDA Human Nutrition Research Center on Aging call these tests "markers" of aging. These researchers believe that they're much more reliable indicators of the age you function at than your age in years. My parents are in their late seventies, but they function as forty-year-olds. They play tennis and golf, swim, lift weights, dance, and party. I look at many of my friends in their forties and see them functioning as seventy-year-olds.

Aerobic power is the most telling measure of your biological age. Followed from year to year, it shows whether or not you are beating Father Time. Unlike the age reflected on your driver's license, your biological age, as measured by aerobic power, can be radically altered. It will change dramatically for the worse through inactivity. By age sixty-five, in both sexes, aerobic power is 40 percent lower than that of young adults if they don't exercise. When I ran my sports science laboratory in Lake Placid, every test subject, regardless of age or athletic ability, was eager to learn his or her maximal aerobic power, or "VO_2 MAX." Under conditions of maximal exertion, VO_2 MAX shows how much oxygen your body can deliver to exercising muscles. The stronger and bigger your heart and lungs, the better conditioned your muscles, and the more red blood cells you have, the higher that number will be. VO_2 MAX is a powerful predictor of athletic performance for runners, cyclists, cross-country skiers, swimmers, and other aerobic athletes. Just as a car's overall horsepower can be measured by computers, so can your horsepower. In fact, VO_2 MAX is easily converted into a horsepower rating.

The toughest aerobic sport of all is Nordic skiing. Athletes in that sport have the highest VO_2 MAX of any athletes in the world. Maurilio DeZolt is one of the best cross-country skiers there is. At the age of forty-three, he led the Italian cross-country ski team to an astounding gold medal at the Lillehammer Olympics in the ten-kilometer relay, beating the scores of the world's best twenty-year-old athletes. He is the ultimate example of turning back the clock, because he was better at forty-three than he was at twenty-three! If you begin training in your twenties, you can continue to get better into your thirties, forties, even fifties. It's never too late. Men can still begin regular aerobic training well into their seventies and see huge improvement. You won't achieve the levels of a person who has exercised all his life, because the heart and lungs will not respond as well to training, but the results will still be substantial.

Muscle is youth. Every decade from age forty you lose up to six pounds of muscle! It may not be apparent, since the size of your arms and legs often remains the same as when you were younger, but fat has replaced muscle. The diagrams show cross sections of the thigh. On the left is the thigh of a twenty-year-old. On the right is the thigh of a seventy-year-old. The seventy-year-old has the same size leg but drastically less muscle and much more fat. Even if your weight stays the same, special computerized X rays show less muscle and more fat with each decade you age. The less muscle you have, the less you can eat without getting fat, since you have less active tissue to burn calories at rest and during exercise. The average twenty-five-year-old man is 18 percent fat, but by age sixty-five he's 38 percent fat! Much of that fat gain is due to the loss of vital, active, calorie-burning muscle.

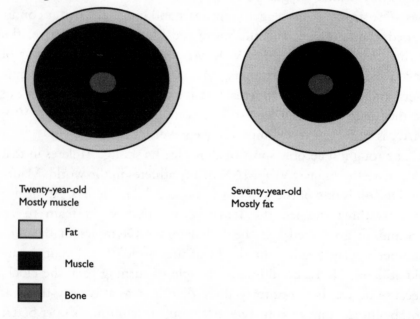

Twenty-year-old
Mostly muscle

Seventy-year-old
Mostly fat

☐ Fat

■ Muscle

▨ Bone

Examine the muscle of aging men under the microscope. Aerobically fit men who don't weight train show the telltale signs of aging with fewer smaller muscle fibers and more scar tissue. But look at the muscle of older men who performed weight training much of their lives. Their muscle looks little different from a twenty-year-old's, concludes Professor Henrik Klitgaard of the August Krogh Institute in Copenhagen, who found robust muscle fibers in older men who weight train. "Endurance training is important, but it won't keep people from getting weak as they get older," he says. No matter how much you run or cycle, remember that two-thirds of your muscle mass is above your hips, untouched by many aerobic exercises. Developing this muscle creates a tremendous engine to roll back the years.

A SPECIAL NOTE TO WOMEN

I hope you'll get this book for your father, brother, husband, or son, but I also hope you'll enjoy it yourself. It has become politically incorrect for men to write books for women, and I won't attempt to cross that boundary here. But in writing and researching this book, every woman I've spoken to expressed a genuine enthusiasm for the material in *Turning Back the Clock,* an advanced knowledge of the concepts of the book, and a real eagerness to try them out. As a group, women are much more knowledgeable about nutrition, sports instruction, and training smart than the men in their lives, perhaps because the pressure to stay young has traditionally been so much higher for women. But since the tables are turning and the pressure is on men to look and act younger, *Turning Back the Clock* can become a tremendous motivational tool for the whole family.

Chapter 2

A Vision of Re-created Youth

I HAVE ONLY A FEW FRIENDS WHO HAVE ALWAYS BEEN EXACTLY WHAT they've wanted to be: muscular enough to have a great physique, trim enough to carry little body fat, energetic enough to rough an expedition anywhere in the world, skilled enough to play most sports well, and mentally tough enough to weather the wildest storm. Like most of my other friends, I just never got around to all of it. I've been in great cardiovascular shape, but was never mistaken for someone with a great body, someone coordinated at sports, or someone dedicated to my personal nutrition. During the last year I've canvassed the best coaches, sports labs, training centers, and spas in America. I've bought a dual-suspension titanium mountain bike, quivers of skis and tennis racquets, dozens of rollerblade frames and mountain bike tires. I've taken every supplement known, from royal jelly to Klamath Lakes Super Blue Green Algae. I've combed scientific literature on training, diet, exercise, and nutrition and interviewed many of the country's best sports scientists.

What I can report to you is that there has been a revolution in food, fitness, and sports technology over the last decade that enables all men to make the physical gains previously open to only a few with either great genetics or amazing dedication. I had never gained a pound of muscle in my life, but put on fourteen pounds of muscle in the last year due to advances in weight training equipment, technique, and nutrition. I can beat kids less than half my age in mountain biking and rollerblading. I've got my body fat down to 8 percent — less than it was when I was a triathlete twenty years ago — without dieting for a single day. My nutrition allows me to do what I want when I want with the energy and vigor of a nineteen-year-old.

At one critical point in every man's life comes the chance to transform himself into precisely what he's always wanted to be. It may be triggered by a heart attack, career disappointment, divorce, middle-age crisis, job loss, or new challenges. But if he grasps that chance, he can become better than he has ever been — stronger, fitter, happier, and more successful — and remain that way for decades. This book presents the power and the opportunity to accomplish just that.

Many men have tried . . . and failed . . . to change themselves by acquiring pop culture's newest habits and behaviors. They lacked a firmly grounded vision of who they should become. By embracing a bold new vision, you can turn back the clock with surprising ease, joy, and speed.

The greatest advances in medicine and science came from neither slow, methodical plodding nor gradual, moderate change. Great advances came in giant leaps made possible only by completely new ways of thinking about problems. The conventional wisdom in the late Middle Ages was that the world was flat. Columbus could set out for the new world only if he was absolutely convinced that the earth was round and had no edges to fall off of. He did so. In modern medicine, the most dramatic bolt-of-lightning breakthroughs also came from men who understood that dramatic solutions come only from fresh, novel visions in which they intensely believe. This is popularly called a new paradigm, and it becomes a blueprint from which we plan and act. To strengthen your resolve, each chapter in this book creates a new paradigm that starkly contrasts with the conventional wisdom.

Psychologically and physically, a true paradigm shift is easier to accomplish and leads to far greater success than minor modifications. How many times have you been truly motivated by someone whose only advice is "everything in moderation"?

Patients of University of California's Dr. Dean Ornish lost more weight and kept it off longer than patients on any other weight program in America. At the same time, their clogged coronary arteries opened without a single medical procedure. How? They rejected the conventional wisdom: eat less to weigh less. They embraced a new paradigm: eat more to weigh less. Dr. Ornish's patients were asked to eat a vegetarian diet. That's a pretty wild change for men who've lived for fifty years on meat and potatoes. What startled Dr. Ornish was that these men found it easier to make a radical change to a super-low-fat vegetarian diet than to make small compromises in their current diet. Moderate changes yield so few positive results that men easily slide back into the comfy lifestyle of their past. But if they make big changes, the changes stick. Why? Because they get immediate results. Rather than making small changes with a promise of good health in the distant future, they make big changes and feel great overnight. In *The Aspern Papers,* Henry James wrote that people "who achieve the miracle of changing their point of view late in life" are "intensely converted." At any age, new paradigms create an intense conversion.

I don't advocate the screaming-through-the-halls kind of misconduct that got me booted from my college dorm, but moderation is nonsense when it comes to achieving terrific health. When the Army says be all you can be, they don't mean there's a gentle hiking path down from the cliff you could take instead of rappelling off the edge. If you want to take a politically correct stab at living longer through moderation, then die moderately young!

In the end, any change practiced over just several weeks will seem routine and ordinary. Why spend the time and effort to incorporate little changes when big changes will accomplish dramatically more, but still appear everyday, ordinary, and livable in the long run? Are American men willing to make big changes? Absolutely. Look at the number who undertake radical reductions in food intake every time they diet. At any given time, 30 percent of men are on diets. They endure a plummeting loss of energy, searing hunger pangs, complete deprivation of any food enjoyment. Men believe in big changes — they've just been sold the wrong changes!

If you lived in the small sugar-producing town of Paia in Maui, your favorite restaurants would serve Japanese, Thai, and vegetarian foods. You would bike to and from work. Your weekend recreation might be six hours of carving and jibing your windsurfer through house-high waves off the Hookipa coast or a mountain bike ride down the Haleakala volcano.

But, you say, I don't live in Hawaii, I live in some postindustrial snake pit where the sun never shines. Well join the club! I live in East Harlem, where there's not a single signpost of the new paradigm. But if you undertake this book as an adventure, you will create your own new dimension right alongside the conventional one. I operate in a southern California dimension alongside the 1954 corporate culture that remains in so many New York midtown and Wall Street firms. I commute on carbon fiber, five-wheeled speed-skating blades, wearing surfing shorts and a Malibu T-shirt. On Wall Street, the "suits" arrive in taxis wearing white shirts, dark clothing, and highly polished shoes. I eat a take-out lunch from California Burrito. The suits eat a heavy meat-and-potatoes lunch. I do my morning reading on an Alpine trainer. The suits read in their offices.

I'm a product of the *Leave It to Beaver* era. I loved coming home from St. Paul's grade school to watch Wally and Beav's latest adventures after brief detours to pack in a five-cent hot fudge sundae at Benslev's and down a half dozen jelly doughnuts at Hazel's Bakery. Friday night, my parents would take me out for a steak-and-french-fry dinner.

So what happened? My paradigm shifted at school in Hanover, New Hampshire, where I discovered a wonderful new life of vigorous physical activity in the great rural New England outdoors. I met Doug Peterson, an Olympic kayaker and cross-country ski racer. Doug seemed like a pretty ordinary guy. It hit me, why can't I be an athlete? I took up rowing, kayaking, and cross-country skiing. The reward for a long hard week in Hanover was a midnight climb up Mt. Moosilauke and a predawn ski down. I fell in love with the feeling of the physical life. I was transformed. I began to pick my foods so I could find ones that made me perform faster or longer. Early evening hikes and bike rides replaced Beav and Wally. Whole-grain breads and cereals replaced sundaes and jelly doughnuts. An afternoon at the Dartmouth skiway or Tuckerman Ravine replaced cruising the streets.

Deepak Chopra wrote in *Ageless Body, Timeless Mind:* "We program our consciousness to a set span of aging, and our biology responds to that programming." Look at that middle-age spread men get in their forties and fifties. Is that genetically programmed? No way! It's the result of misguided nutrition and physical training. Why? Because the psychologically programmed paradigm for aging is the expectation that we look and behave in a different manner with each passing decade. We're comfortable in the paradigm that urges us to let go of our youth and embrace a sedentary middle age. Men accept culturally programmed senescence. Society expects us to look, behave, and perform in a peculiar "middle-aged" way in our forties, fifties, and sixties. Many of us just get with the program. We surrender our physique, power, potency, strength, and endurance to the expectations of society. Recent research shows that for those who have switched paradigms, there is no middle age. By changing the paradigm to that of Teddy Roosevelt, who carried youth and vigor with him all the days of his life, we can brag to our grandchildren, "We're just a bunch of kids with outdated birth certificates."

As you assemble your new paradigm, try to create a brilliant, guiding vision of who you hope to become. That process is called imagery. You may think of imagery as some New Age trend soon to fall by the wayside. Yet most men use imagery every day. We provoke anxiety, doom, and gloom when we imagine getting fired, being rejected by co-workers, or failing to finish a project. That imagery is so potent it can cause ulcers, high blood pressure, even heart disease. So why don't we use imagery for peaceful purposes? No one ever taught us how! Imagery is what ties all the pieces together. Imagery is what allows men to imagine the future, create a plan for it, and live it.

We can envision and imagine catastrophe, but we don't create a bold and imaginative vision of who we think we are, who we think we can be, and what we think we can do. With the help of this book, I hope you'll create a dynamic picture of who you want to be as a physical being, which will give you the power, energy, and enthusiasm to transform yourself. Try each night as you fall asleep imagining yourself as leaner, more muscular, more graceful. Practice a dramatic ski racing turn or tennis attack in your mind. At first, you'll see little. But rather than forcing yourself to see a technicolor film on the first try, take the advice of New York psychiatrist Dr. Arthur Phillips. Keep it low key. Just say to yourself, Okay, if I could see a new ski turn, what would it look like. That kind of suggestive language makes bold, vivid images appear from nowhere. Imaging expert Martin Rossman, M.D., the co-director of the Academy for Guided Imagery in Mill Valley, California, has an excellent series of books and tapes that can help you further your imaging skills. Dr. Lee Pulos of Adventures in Learning in Vancouver, B.C., has created a wonderful series of tapes for sports-specific performance. The power of the imagination is the ability to recall and use images in real-life situations. When you're pumping iron, bring to life that image of yourself as stronger and leaner. When you're called on to make a presentation, see yourself as a powerful, dynamic figure. Build your self-image so you become the new paradigm of youth and vigor.

Chapter 3

Be an Athlete

"WANNA COME OUT AND PLAY?" EVER REFUSE THAT OFFER AS A KID? NOT likely. Nothing was beyond the imagination. After some negotiation with your playmates, you could be Batman, Robin Hood, or General Patton. The toys were awesome, from hula hoops and potato-shooting spud guns to Lionel train sets. Well, you have that same opportunity to play today. Sport is play. Kevlar rollerblades, carbon fiber bikes, and fiberglass skating skis are the new toys. You still get to dress up and play in a world of make-believe. You can ride a Greg LeMond racing bike, play with Sampras's tennis racquet, hit with Arnold Palmer's golf clubs, or ski on Jean-Claude Killy's slalom boards. Sport is a great fantasy world. You should learn how to play again. It was the best fun as a kid, and it's the best fun as a grown-up.

Most of us feel a false obligation to subtract one pleasure after the other from life, plying the predawn darkness practicing an exercise we hate, giving up the meals we love, tossing aside the drink we enjoy. Help! There's got to be a reward! There is! That reward is looking, feeling, and acting like an athlete in a sport you grow to love. You might look at me slightly cross-eyed and say: I can't be an athlete, I'm overweight, ungainly, hopelessly out of shape, or was never picked to play sports in school. Well, join the club! No one ever considered me or any of my friends for traditional American sports like basketball, baseball, football, or hockey. That's true of about 95 percent of Americans! My brothers called me a natural klutz. But at age fifteen, an exercise physiologist took me aside and said, "Look, you have the build and skills to be a really great bike racer, runner, or skier." I took up all three sports that year.

At forty-seven I still compete and win at a variety of different sports, from mountain biking to speed skating and cross-country skiing. I still get creamed in lots of other sports, but do them for the true love of the sport. As we move into the twenty-first century, I predict that more and more Americans will take their reward from sports rather than alcohol, junk food, cigarettes, and drugs. In places like Boulder, Colorado; Hanover, New Hampshire; Paia, Maui; and Stowe, Vermont, great sports are already the reward after a long day at the office, not a beer and a burger. It's a much purer high with tremendous long-term psychological, medical, and physical payoffs.

You may be hard-pressed to believe it, but I'm not alone in saying how much better I feel after a good bike ride, tennis game, or gym workout than after a glass of wine or a bottle of beer. That powerful feeling of being an athlete makes me much more productive and allows me to work or play far longer and harder.

Conventional Wisdom:
Walk, crawl, paddle in the pool, just so long as it's dull.
New Paradigm:
Be an athlete! Sports-improvement technology and rapid skill advancement can quickly unleash the hidden athlete in you.

Even if you look like Mr. Magoo, trapped somewhere in that low-key, slump-shouldered frame lurks real athletic talent. Everyone has athletic talent. When I ran my sports science center for the Winter Olympics teams in Lake Placid, I had the opportunity to visit secret laboratories in East Germany and the old Soviet Union. Their sports science centers selected individuals for specific sports. They had very exacting methods that examined heart size, lung power, muscle type, bone structure, and over two hundred physical skills.

Curiously, they found a wide range of athletic talents that differed significantly from one individual to the next. There was no one "natural athlete."

At our own laboratory, we were very impressed that virtually everyone who came to us for testing, identified as an "athlete" or not, had genuine athletic talent, from overweight French dairy farmers to sedentary Manhattan executives. One man might have a ski racer's low center of gravity, knock-knees, pigeon-toes, and sprint muscle, while another might have a marathoner's long legs, narrow hips, and endurance muscle. Some had hair-trigger reaction time or great sports vision, even though they had no visible athletic endowment. My conclusion is this: the average "nonathlete" has been badly cheated by a physical education system that selects very few for a very narrow range of sports. That's the bad news. The good news is that it's never too late to start playing the sport that's right for you! If for no other reason, pick a new sport to spite that high school gym teacher who thought you were a loser.

Take great pride in continually improving your skills, endurance, speed, power, and ability against your own personal standard and within your own physiology. You can create your own enthusiasm and excitement by the objective progress you measure. When you do look around, I bet you'll be surprised how really good you are. The more you look and feel like an athlete, the more you will want to transform yourself into a bold, vigorous, and dynamic person. The process of becoming an athlete can give you a new identity. Your posture will improve, your skin will assume a more healthy glow, and your stride will quicken.

"Great," you're saying. "Who the hell does this guy think he's talking about? Face reality. I'm over the hill. How can I possibly keep up with a twenty-year-old?" One approach is to create a level playing field by getting into a new, even obscure sport where there are no experts. Exploit the developing technology to get a clear, cutting-edge advantage, then take what you've learned from other sports and apply them. My friends ran marathons in the mid-1970s before the big crest, then got out. In the early 1980s they took up windsurfing and Iron Man contests. Once triathlons became a regular part of the country club circuit, they ducked out for mountain bike racing, speed skating, winter sport triathlons, Nordic skiing, and snowboarding in a never-ending quest to stay at the front of the pack for as many years as possible.

Following a late-breaking AIDS scare, one of our edit rooms displayed a cartoon of a cross-eyed fairly geeky-looking college student with Coke-bottle-lens glasses. The best-looking girls on campus are surrounding him, swooning. The caption reads: "Gee, I've never had a date." If you weren't a top college, professional, or Olympic athlete or you are even a newcomer to fitness altogether, I want you! Chances are you have virgin joints with little wear and tear. You have spectacular amounts of improvement to undergo and a remarkable long-term future as an athlete. Virtually any suggestion made in this book will yield quick and easy results.

"Hey! Yo! You out in left field. Move a little farther left." I did as the coach instructed me in baseball. Another boy moved into the main left-field position for practice at Camp Wyanoke in Wolfeboro, New Hampshire. I was moved out of place just in case the ball ever actually came my direction. Most kids would have been insulted, perhaps crushed, to be a backup left fielder. I wasn't. I knew I couldn't touch the ball, never mind catch it. I'm not going to mislead you into believing I'm any great athlete. In fact my junior high and high school teachers thought I was the sorriest excuse for an athlete that had come down the line in a very long time. But that's the credential I'd like to use: Bob Arnot, not-a-natural-athlete. I am a completely constructed athlete. Not a single motion comes "naturally" to me. So why bother to read a chapter on how to be much, much better at sports from someone who's not a natural athlete? The proof that *Turning Back the Clock* really works is in the klutz who became an athlete by taking the best from the newly developing field of sports science.

But many men claim they just don't have the energy, stamina, or strength to become an athlete. It is my firm conviction that these men practice poor nutrition. I believe that over 70 percent of a man's ability to exercise vigorously and grow new muscle is tied to the foods he eats. That's why the first major section of this book is on Eating Young. By following the guidelines in these chapters, you will find becoming an athlete a real joy.

EATING YOUNG

Chapter 4

Feedforward Eating

DO YOU EAT IN DESPERATION? DO YOU PUSH FOOD DOWN IN HOPES OF drowning fatigue, depression, and mental fogginess? Does hunger drive you to the vending machine, doughnut shop, or hamburger stand despite your best intentions? If so, you've become a slave. How? By allowing TV commercials, magazine ads, fast-food billboards, and the sight and smell of food to drive primitive centers in your lower brain to tell you what and when to eat.

Foods can be powerful medicines that control how we look, feel, and perform. We can lose fat, grow muscle, gain energy, and vanquish hunger through the proper selection of foods and timing of meals. By eating the right foods, cranking back the clock becomes easy and fun.

Conventional Wisdom:
Listen to your body.
New Paradigm:
Seize control of your mind and body through the foods you eat.

Rat behavior is controlled through "feedback" eating. Good rats learn quickly that they will be rewarded with food for correctly performing a task. Many humans are trained like laboratory rats to reward themselves with food. They wait for fatigue, hunger, elation, depression, weakness, sleepiness, or anxiety to tell them when to eat, then reward themselves with high-fat, high-sugar foods. Eating becomes a game of never-ending catch-up where you respond to the moment rather than devising eating tactics for a far more success-ful day.

Allowing food to run your life this way is crazy! What if we waited until a car's fuel tank was empty before we filled the tank with more gas? Highways would be strewn with abandoned cars. In most other aspects of our lives, we plan in advance, but when it comes to eating, we let Mother Nature or Madison Avenue do the driving.

Feedforward eating is consuming the right foods in advance of a meeting, a workout, a nap, or concentrated intellectual effort so that you feel and perform exactly as you want. With feedforward eating, you plan your day by how you would like to feel at a given time or for a specific activity. You then eat foods that will make you feel the way you want at the time you require. Need to be more aggressive and alert for a big morning meeting? No problem. Want to recover faster from a tough workout? Easy! Need to relax and concentrate? Kid stuff. Want to feel more energetic during your evening workout? Done. In the old paradigm, you were a slave to food. In the new paradigm, you eat before the sight and smell of food or the pangs of hunger manipulate you to make poor food choices. In feedback eating our senses tell us what to eat. We stop eating because we feel full. We start eating because we feel hungry. Feedback eating relies on primitive senses common to many lower forms of life. Feed-forward eating relies on real intellect.

On a feedback day, you wake up at 6:30 A.M. famished. You grab a bagel and a cup of coffee, then run out the door for your big pre-sentation at the quarterly meeting. Halfway through the event, your blood sugar crashes. You fumble for words, your performance falls flat. Deflated and depressed, you drown your despair in a big glass of cola and a cinnamon twist doughnut. You're rewarded with fifteen minutes of feeling marginally better. By the time you answer your boss's summons in regard to your less-than-stunning performance, your blood sugar has crashed and burned. You wobble back and forth in her office painting a picture of gloom and doom.

For lunch you eat a big bowl of pasta with two slices of french bread. You sit down to work on next year's budget, but you're so sleepy you can only crawl through January and February before grinding to a halt. You head to the gym for a workout, but fifteen minutes into a StairMaster climb, your legs are rubbery, your pace slows, and you quit. For dinner you eat a big piece of meat, have a salad with lots of blue cheese dressing, and a big glass of milk. After work, you hit the sack after an exhausting and unnerving day but toss and turn for hours, unable to fall asleep. By 6:30 A.M. you're tired and haggard, ill prepared to face another day. The foods you ate weren't all so terrible, but how you used them was a disaster. So what do you do?

1. Resign.
2. Wait for a demotion.
3. Inquire at personnel about early retirement.
4. Resolve to begin feedforward eating.

On a feedforward day, you wake up at 6:30 A.M. relaxed and refreshed from a great night's sleep. For breakfast you have whole-grain cereal with skim milk. Your metabolism climbs steadily. The protein makes you alert. The whole grains keep your blood sugar at a steady, high-performance level. At the presentation you feel alert and confident, on top of the world. Your less-wide-awake colleagues are awed by your commanding presence and coherency at this hour of the morning. Your boss congratulates you after the meeting. You plan your lunch as a preworkout meal so that you can exercise at your best. You have chicken and lots of slow-burning carbohydrates. The protein keeps you alert for a harried afternoon. The slow-burning carbos prevent a crash and burn. In the gym, you're stoked. Every minute on the StairMaster is better than the one before. You move to the weight room, where you feel a tremendous pump at the end of each set. You leave relaxed and refreshed. You drink a protein-carbohydrate sports beverage to speed muscle building and refuel your muscles for another great workout tomorrow. For dinner, you go light on the protein and stock up on lots of slow-burning carbohydrates like oatmeal, black beans, or pure whole-grain breads. When bedtime comes, you're out like a light. At 6:30 A.M., you're ready to rock and roll again.

There it is. Practice feedback eating and you eat from a position of weakness. Primitive senses tell you it's time to eat by triggering alarms. When you respond to those alarms, you'll overeat, since it takes ten to thirty minutes to feel the calming or energizing effect of foods. Practice feedforward eating by using the high-level intelligence of the human brain to plan how you want to feel and act with the precision of a laser-guided missile.

DAILY BENEFITS OF FEEDFORWARD EATING

Alertness

Defense Department–sponsored research labs are now conducting studies on a specific amino acid, tyrosine, that keeps concentration high over twelve hours for top jet fighter pilots. The armed forces are also experimenting with choline to extend endurance. You can achieve the same effect by increasing the protein in a meal relative to the amount of carbohydrate. Do you have an important meeting or presentation? Are you about to go work out? Then increased protein intake makes sense. Branched-chain amino acids such as leucine during exercise may increase alertness and increase the time until you fatigue. But eat a late-night protein meal and find yourself staring at the ceiling counting sheep for hours.

Relaxation

When you can't unwind at home in the evening, feel anxious and cranky with the kids, increase the carbohydrate content of your meal and decrease the protein. But if you eat lots of carbos before a big presentation, expect to be dull as doughnuts.

Recovery

Just finished working out? Now is the time for a good hit of protein. If you like simple or refined sugars, now's the time to eat them, too. Your recovery will be stunningly faster with this combination.

New Muscle

Are you a hard gainer who never seems to put on any muscle mass? You can increase your body's drive to build new muscle by eating larger quantities of special foods around your workout.

Fat Loss

You can lose fat simply by changing the foods that you eat. What foods? Slow-burning carbohydrates will steady your blood sugar. Faster-burning carbos are like shooting fat into your veins and aiming them at the roll around the middle of your belly. You can drop five to ten pounds just by changing carbohydrates.

Increased Potency

New recovery drinks increase the amount of the male sex hormone testosterone available to the body after exercise. They also help increase muscle mass and decrease body fat. That combination further increases the amount of testosterone available to increase potency.

Smother Free Radicals

Free radicals zap your body millions of times a day, increasing your risk of cancer and heart disease. Doctors theorize that free radicals cause cholesterol to become a harmful substance that narrows arteries, leading to heart disease. By eating foods that are high in antioxidants, you can smother free radicals. When you exercise vigorously, you create lots of free radicals, but if you take antioxidants during exercise or right after, you reverse this effect. You can also reverse the effect of bad environments, like the San Diego Freeway or the city of Los Angeles, that make lots of free radicals.

Play Longer

The advent of technical sports drinks and sports bars allows the average mortal to play longer, better, and faster. By planning to take these foods before you feel wobbly and crash, you'll put in a seamless performance.

More Power

The ability to play really hard depends on fully stocked muscle fuel depots. You can stock those fuel stores chock full of energy by eating the right kinds of carbos and proteins at exactly the proper time.

No Pain

"No pain, no gain" refers to athletes who make countless fueling and nutritional errors. Eat right and train smart for spectacular gains without the pain. Much of the pain comes from working out when you're really thin on fuel.

LONG-TERM BENEFITS OF FEEDFORWARD EATING

You Are What You Ate

The body you have today is built almost entirely from what you have eaten over the last six months. "If the proteins you eat are of poor quality, then all the structures of your body, muscles, bones, blood, teeth, and pinkies will be poor quality," says Dr. Michael Colgan, the director of the Colgan Institute, a nutritional analysis group in San Diego. The dearth of first-rate nutrients results in weak muscles, poor bone quality, second-rate tendons and joints, miserly energy stores, and even poor-quality fat stored in the worst places.

Less Fat

More of the right foods increases your metabolism so you can lose weight. The old paradigm of low-calorie meals failed abysmally with a 90 percent–plus failure rate. Why? These dieters destroyed the thing that could help them keep weight off: lean muscle mass. In fact at least 40 percent of all they lost was lean muscle!

A Young Immune System

A bulletproof immune system can decrease your risk of minor illnesses from colds to flus and major illnesses from cancer to heart disease. A strong immune system speeds recovery, which means faster progress in aerobic or weight training. Many researchers believe that aging is a declining immune system. A strong immune system slows aging.

More Muscle

Real gains in muscle mass are possible only with cutting-edge nutrition. The right high-quality proteins can speed the development of strong, young muscle.

Chapter 5

Control Your Blood Sugar

RALPH HAS A DIRTY LITTLE SECRET. ONCE A WILD RECREATIONAL USER OF heroin, cocaine, and alcohol, he's now become a sugar junkie. Each evening, in the anonymity of his home, Ralph withdraws four pints of frozen yogurt from the refrigerator. After consuming the third pint he's flying. His blood sugar level has been launched into the stratosphere. Still, he shovels the last pint into his mouth to keep his sugar high as long as possible before the terrible crash. Like millions of Americans, he's addicted to massive amounts of sugar and processed foods. It's his last addiction and the only one he can't break.

Sugar, he says, is a really crummy drug. "A sugar high is uncontrollable with a high discomfort value. It's really just a buzz . . . nothing special about it." In his worst periods of sugar addiction, he is angry, hostile, depressed, fatigued, and fat. He can put eight pounds on in just four days.

Ralph's case lies at the extreme end of a spectrum of abuse widely practiced by American men.

Conventional Wisdom:
Controlling blood sugar is for people with diabetes.

New Paradigm:

Control your blood sugar and you control your weight, mental energy, physical endurance, and hunger.

Picture a car engine getting fuel in huge spurts. With each spurt, the car engine roars to life, throwing you back in your seat, but then it coughs, sputters, and nearly comes to a halt. The cycle is repeated over and over until you turn green and nauseous. Now picture a huge turbine jet engine with exquisite fuel-control devices that deliver a steady, even flow of fuel and a powerful ride so smooth you feel motionless. That's the difference between crash-and-burn eating and eating that steadies your blood sugar.

WHY STEADY YOUR BLOOD SUGAR?

Decrease Belly Fat

I couldn't for the life of me lose the last little bit of "fat around the belly" last year. I undertook the knee-jerk reaction of most men who train in aerobic sports: I simply worked out longer and harder while eating less food. It didn't work. Why? I was trapped in a vicious cycle of eating bulk quantities of highly refined white flour disguised as what I believed to be healthy, even athletic, foods such as bagels, pastas, breads, and cereals. Large quantities of refined white flours and simple sugars have a common effect. They can cause large in-creases in blood sugar, raising it from a fasting level as low as 70 to 180 or higher! This signals the body to store fat around your belly. Why? The high levels of blood sugar trigger your body to release excess amounts of the hormone insulin. Each time a high blood sugar level triggers a large release of insulin, excess calories are turned into fat, which is, by preference, stored around your belly. This belly fat is the worst place to store fat, since it poses the highest risk for heart disease.

Once I stopped eating refined flours and simple sugars, my belly fat vanished in a matter of weeks without any serious attempt to diet.

31

Controlling blood sugar is one of the vanishingly few "tricks" there are to force your body to shed fat. The body doesn't need high levels of blood sugar and functions much better on the steady, moderate level that whole grains, beans, and fruits and vegetables deliver. Excess blood sugar simply spills over into fat.

Cut Hunger

One prominent reason men get hungry between meals is a rapid fall in blood sugar brought on by large quantities of simple sugars or highly processed foods, especially when combined with caffeine, alcohol, or tobacco. Try this. Have a bagel or several pieces of toast for breakfast. Eat enough to satiate your hunger. Now see if you're not ravenously hungry by late morning. Research has shown that by eating foods that make your blood sugar rise and fall quickly, you will eat more calories at your next meal. How many? At least 300. I found this out the hard way. After my morning workout at the gym, I'd take a large sugary carbohydrate replacement beverage. Boom! One hour later I was ravenous. I ingested four slices of turkey, four ears of corn, two giant pieces of cornbread, stuffing, even gravy! I was so hungry I couldn't control my intake less than one hour after consuming 750 calories! However, if I maintained a steady, moderate blood sugar level, I could control precisely what I wanted to eat: salad, vegetables, fruits, and whole grains. When I'm really hungry, I just lose control. Doughnuts, cake, and ice cream are all fair game. I just can't eat enough. Controlling your blood sugar is a great example of feedforward eating. Don't spike your blood sugar and you'll be able to pick and choose foods that are really good for you. Pop your blood sugar and your appetite will spin out of control.

End Fatigue and Burnout

Day-long crash-and-burn eating can cause your adrenal glands to release lots of adrenaline and stress hormones. Those stress hormones do you nothing but harm if you blast your body and brain with them time and time again during the day, especially with caffeine added to the mix. You'll be tired, worn out, and unhappy.

Cliff Sheats, author of *Lean Bodies,* believes that you can cause the adrenal glands to tire, creating a chronic-fatigue-like syndrome. He's had good luck with fatigue patients with a diet that doesn't cause big bursts of blood sugar.

End Wrecked Workouts

How many times have you "bonked" during a workout because your blood sugar fell into the sewer? "Bonking," for the uninitiated, is when your brain feels like the power has been pulled and your legs turn to rubber. Reduced, refined, and concentrated sugars have an erratic effect on blood sugar levels. Unless you carefully control your intake of foods that raise blood sugar levels abruptly, your workouts are prone to disaster. The effect is even more devastating during competition. I remember watching a top U.S. skater throw away her gold medal by gulping down pure honey before her final Olympic performance. She simply crashed when her blood sugar level collapsed halfway through her routine. A stable blood sugar level during exercise increases workout output and prolongs the time you can play until exhaustion hits.

Slow Out-of-Control Aging

People with diabetes who have continually high blood sugar levels run into terrible long-term complications. High levels may destroy their hearts, eyes, kidneys, and limbs. One theory is that high blood sugar levels destroy the body's connective tissue. Researchers on aging speculate that ordinary mortals who artificially keep their blood sugars high by eating massive amounts of processed foods hasten the aging process.

Cut Mental Fatigue

Low blood sugar can cause fatigue so profound that it's just not possible to concentrate on the mundane mental chores of daily living. This is most noticeable in crash-and-burn eaters who don't eat at all after they burn. They have a bagel and coffee for breakfast. To avoid gaining weight, they avoid eating after their blood sugar has plummeted at midmorning. By lunch they can barely see straight to get to the company cafeteria.

Boost Nutrients

Most foods that increase blood sugar are nutritionally bankrupt. That goes not just for soft drinks and hard candies, but also for many products made with white flour. Replacing them with whole grains, fruits, and vegetables adds high doses of thousands of energy-enhancing, body-building, and disease-preventing nutrients.

HOW TO STEADY YOUR BLOOD SUGAR

Eat Slow-Burning Carbos

Slow-burning carbohydrates keep blood sugar in a healthy range because they are absorbed slowly enough from the intestine into the bloodstream so that there is no fast rise in blood sugar. They maintain steady, healthy blood sugar that will give you a constant level of mental and physical energy. Slow carbos are whole foods that contain a powerful package of carbohydrate, vitamins, minerals, protein, and fiber. They should comprise the majority of the calories that you eat. A change from fast to slow carbos made me feel great from the first day I switched. Slow carbos are a central part of any weight-reduction strategy because they keep you from becoming hungry between meals and prevent the spike in blood sugar that can cause fat around the belly. You'll find that on slow carbos, you really don't have the hunger you would otherwise have.

Here's an example: Have a large serving of oatmeal with whole wheat toast and low-fat milk for breakfast. Your intestine will slowly and steadily feed sugar into your bloodstream. You won't get the thirty-second "Oh my God I'm alive again" sort of hit that Morning Thunder delivers. However, by the time you're out the door in the morning, your blood sugar will be headed for a nice healthy range where it will remain for as many as four hours. You'll be more even tempered, less hungry, and have all the energy you need for a good morning of work or play. Even at lunch, your blood sugar will remain thirty to forty points over fasting, just where you want it. This allows you to make healthy choices at lunch, uninfluenced by mental craving or searing pit-of-the-stomach hunger.

The opposite will occur if you have a cola with a bagel. You'd get a big blood sugar spike, crash within an hour, and then find that mental and physical fatigue set in over the course of the next several hours. Many men think that they suffer from the ravages of aging or a chronic fatigue syndrome when in fact they just eat poorly. My father, who has practiced psychiatry for fifty years, has treated innumerable patients for depression and fatigue when the major contributing factor to their ill health was a terrible diet.

Here are the very best slow-burning carbohydrates. They should comprise at least 70 percent of what you eat.

Cereals: grits, oatmeal, oatbran cereal, wheat germ, and whole-grain cooked cereals.

Legumes: dried beans; baked beans; black-eyed peas; kidney, pinto, and navy beans; lentils; and split peas.

Whole grains: barley, wheat bulgur, quinoa, amaranth, and millet.

Vegetables: lima beans, peas, artichokes, asparagus, beans, beets, broccoli, and tomatoes.

Avoid Fast Sugars

Fast sugars are carbohydrates that are quickly absorbed from the intestine into the bloodstream, causing a sharp rise in blood sugar. Fast sugars are the hallmark of the reactive eater. When blood sugar sinks after a sharp rise, hunger appears, as does fatigue. Reactive eaters instinctively reach for more fast-burning sugars and are doomed to repeat a cycle throughout the day of blood sugar levels that surge and crash. The use of fast carbos is usually the result of poor planning. With slow-burning carbos, it's unlikely you'll need fast carbos. Fast carbos have little fiber, vitamins, minerals, or protein. Here are the fast sugars to avoid: white-flour products such as white bread, pancakes, bagels, and cereals; soft drinks; desserts; muffins and doughnuts; and candy bars made with fast sugars.

Now you may say, "Hey, wait a minute, Dr. Bob, I thought I ate lots of complex carbohydrates, but you say bagels and pastas aren't healthy foods. How come?" Many men are fooled into believing that all pastas, grains, bagels, and cereals are good, healthy, complex carbohydrates. In fact many of them are white-flour products that, to my way of thinking, aren't much better than eating sugar with vitamin pills. In fact white bread will raise your blood sugar higher and faster than table sugar and at the same rate as a Mars bar!

Do fast sugars have a place? Specially constructed fast sugars can be used during and immediately after prolonged exercise precisely because they do work so quickly. Taking fast-acting carbs as fuel during and immediately after exercise is their best legitimate use.

Sugar is the great nutritional enticer and can be used for good as well as evil purposes. Sprinkled on a fatty cinnamon bun, it tricks the body into eating massive amounts of terrible food without ever producing satiety. However, using sugar on a whole-grain cereal or oatmeal as a way of enticing you to eat really healthy foods is just fine. A teaspoon of sugar is a meager fifteen calories. I'd far rather eat a terrific cereal with a little sugar sprinkled on it than a cereal that has masses of corn syrup embedded in it. Fifteen calories of cane sugar on a 300-calorie bowl of oatmeal won't really affect your blood sugar and is a perfectly reasonable practice.

Balance Every Meal

Simple sugars and heavily processed foods aren't the only foods that can cause your blood sugar to rise rapidly. Research measurements show that terrific foods like carrots, parsnips, and cornflakes may have the same devastating effect on your blood sugar as a candy bar. You can avoid that fast release of sugar from your intestine into your bloodstream by eating other foods that release sugar more slowly. The best way to plan meals is to be certain that you have slow-burning carbos to counteract any fast-burning sugars.

David Jenkins, M.D., Ph.D., of the University of Toronto, popularized this concept, calling it the Glycemic Index. Dr. Jenkins actually measured the rise in blood sugar in response to individual foods tested one at a time. The higher the position of the food in the following table, the more likely your blood sugar will soar when you eat it. At the top of the list is glucose, which causes your blood sugar to double. At the bottom are soybeans and lentils. The reason for making certain that foods at the top of the list are mixed with foods at the bottom is simple. You wouldn't make a fire in a fireplace with just newspapers. You'd have to stand there for hours just throwing in one Sunday *Times* after another to keep the heat going. But if you add slow-burning logs at the same time, you'll have a nice even-burning fire. That's exactly what you want from food, a nice even-burning fire. The list of foods on the next page, which appeared in the *Journal of Sports Sciences* in 1991, is ranked from high to low using the Glycemic Index constructed by Dr. Ed Coyle of the University of Texas at Austin. The quantities listed are needed to obtain fifty grams of carbohydrate.

Some scientists now scoff at the use of the Glycemic Index because they say all meals mix foods of different glycemic values so that the overall effect is produced by the combined values of the foods in the meal. For anyone who eats picture-perfect meals from the Department of Agriculture's handbook, that combined value will be nearly perfect. But for men who eat from vending machines, or eat meals and snacks largely composed of refined white flours, simple sugars, and foods at the high end of the scale, the result will be a meal that causes the blood sugar level to soar. White-flour pizza with a cola and a cookie will blast your blood sugar clear through the ozone layer. An ideal meal or snack will always contain some fiber and at least an ounce of protein.

Eat Fiber with Every Meal

The more fiber you eat from whole grains, vegetables, and fruits, the slower sugar is absorbed into the blood from the intestine. Fiber also slows the absorption of carbohydrates from the intestine into the bloodstream. That reduces blood sugar levels after meals and reduces insulin concentrations. By taking more fiber, even with foods high on the Glycemic Index scale, you slow the blood sugar rise they would otherwise create. The best fibers to keep blood sugar levels

Food	Amount for 50 Grams Carbohydrate
High-Glycemic	
Sugars	
Glucose	4.2 tbsp
Sucrose (white granular)	4.2 tbsp
Sucrose (white powdered)	6.6 tbsp
Syrups/jellies	
Cane and maple syrup	3.9 tbsp
Corn syrup (light)	3.4 tbsp
Honey	2.8 tbsp
Molasses (medium)	4.2 tbsp
Beverages	
6% sucrose solution	3.5 cups
7.5% maltodextrin and sugar	2.8 cups
10% corn syrup (carbonated drink)	2.1 cups
20% maltodextrin solution	1.1 cups
Cereal products	
Bagel (2 oz each)	1.6 bagels
Bread (white or whole meal, 1 oz slice)	3.5 slices
Bread sticks	6.7 sticks
Cornflakes	2 cups
Fruits	
Raisins	0.41 cup
Vegetables	
Potato (baked, 7 oz)	1 potato
Potato (boiled and mashed)	1.5 cups
Sweet corn (yellow)	1.2 cups
Moderate-Glycemic	
Cereal products	
Oatmeal	2.1 cups, cooked
Rice	1 cup, cooked
Spaghetti, macaroni	1.5 cups, cooked
Whole-grain rye bread (1 oz slice)	3.5 slices
Fruits	
Grapes (American slip skin)	3.1 cups
Grapes (European)	1.8 cups
Orange (navel, 5 oz each)	3 oranges

Food	Amount for 50 Grams Carbohydrate
Vegetables	
Corn (yellow, boiled)	1.2 cups
Yams (boiled or baked)	1.3 cups of cubes
Legumes	
Baked beans	0.9 cup
Low-Glycemic	
Fruits	
Apple (raw, 5 oz)	2.4 medium apples
Applesauce (sweetened)	1 cup
Cherries (sweet, raw)	44 cherries
Dates (dried)	8 dates
Figs (raw, 2 oz)	5 figs
Grapefruit (raw, 4 oz)	2.5 grapefruits
Peach (raw, 3 oz)	5 peaches
Pear (raw, 6 oz)	2 pears
Plum (raw, 2 oz)	5.6 plums
Legumes	
Butter beans	1.4 cups
Chickpeas	1.1 cups
Green beans	1.7 cups
Green peas	2.1 cups
Kidney beans	1.2 cups
Navy beans	1.1 cups
Red lentils	1.2 cups
Dairy Products	
Skim milk	4.2 cups
Whole milk	4.4 cups
Yogurt (plain custard)	2.8 cups

down are soluble fibers and include high-quality breakfast cereals, whole grains, and beans. These are best included in every meal and snack.

Eat Vegetarian

Vegetarians naturally eat meals that create extremely even blood sugar levels, which may be why they appear so mellow. I'm convinced that the reason they feel so good is that they eat so little processed food, simple sugar, or animal fat. I'm not convinced that they feel any better than nonvegetarians who do the same. Nonetheless, Dr. Dean Ornish, director and president of the Preventive Medicine Research Institute at the University of California, San Francisco, has observed that his heart patients feel so good so fast on a vegetarian diet that they're far more willing to stay on it than on a diet simply lower in fat.

Get Fit

If you're out of shape and overweight, your body responds sluggishly to insulin. In response to high blood sugar, your body will make even more insulin, which can make you even fatter and more unhealthy. However, a regular program of aerobic exercise will increase your body's ability to respond to insulin so that your body need not make as much of it. Fit men make less insulin when they eat fast sugars than unfit men. Experts refer to this phenomenon as metabolic fitness, since fit men are less likely to have big swings in their blood sugar level and can more easily tolerate heavy loads of sugar. The best way to get an extra buzz from food is with regular exercise.

Practice Hunger Prophylaxis

I'm a big believer in preventing the mad scramble to the vending machine. How? Stockpile your own slow-burning snacks. I keep a drawer full of foods that combine fiber, protein, and slow-burning carbohydrates. The ones I keep in the office are Parrillo Bars, Clif Bars, and Fantastic Foods products. I'll have one of these complete minimeal snacks between meals.

Flatten the Tail

If you do eat foods that cause your sugar to reach very high levels and you aren't going to stop, you may want to consider slowing the subsequent fall of blood sugar. Techies call this "flattening the tail," meaning that the line on the graph showing a fall in blood sugar is long and flat instead of steeply descending and short. If you don't read graphs, that simply means you don't have a big drop. I "flatten the tail" after drinking a high-sugar sports drink like Opti Fuel 2 or Hydra Fuel. So I don't crash, I'll have foods that are slow-burning carbos such as lentil soup or black-eyed peas within sixty minutes after the sports drink. For me, that flattens the tail for the entire afternoon so that I'm not hungry at all. On days that I've waited for the crash, I've eaten 1,500 calories more than I wanted to by the time the day is out.

Eat Breakfast

A normal man's blood sugar on rising is about 70. That's too low on which to do much serious thinking or exercise. It will naturally tend to come up on its own, but only slowly over the course of several hours after you get out of bed in the morning. Breakfast brings your blood sugar up quickly, setting the pattern for the rest of your day. Coffee and toast are like throwing a newspaper and lighter fluid into the fire. You'll get a quick pop and then suffer the consequences of falling blood sugar. I'll have oatmeal with skim milk or a high-fiber cereal with milk or an egg-white-only omelette with low-fat cheese and whole wheat toast. Each of these three breakfast selections gets me to lunch with lots of energy and little hunger. Performance on standard tests of proficiency, reaction time, and recall all suffer in men who don't eat breakfast.

Fix Your Addiction to Sugar Highs

Stabilizing blood sugar levels by eating regular meals that have fiber, protein, and slow-burning carbohydrates is the best start to fixing a sugar addiction. Alcoholics are highly prone to a sugar addiction because they have such awful eating habits. The best immediate fix is a big breakfast with high-quality protein and slow-burning carbos to get you through the morning. If you follow the other guidelines in this chapter, you'll find beating a sugar addiction much easier to do.

There's little surprise that recovering alcoholics like Ralph crave sugar. He can erase depression, anxiety, hunger, fatigue, and shakiness with a big boost of sugar even if it's for a fleetingly short time. He'd do far better to beat depression, anxiety, hunger, and fatigue by eating slow carbos throughout the day.

Summary. My own experience with steadying blood sugar has been very positive. I have been caught walking the halls of CBS News by everyone from Dan Rather to Paula Zahn with candy bars, cookies, and Twinkies. You name it I ate it. Steadying my blood sugar has given me terrific control over what I eat. Since I'm just not as hungry, I can pick and choose among great foods. I don't crash during exercise anymore, nor do I crave sweets. My body fat is the lowest since high school. It did take several months to break my own addiction to sugar highs, but I'm glad I did. I don't completely avoid fast sugars, but when I do eat them, I eat enough slow burners to mellow them out.

I've made "Control Your Blood Sugar" the first food chapter because it makes the other steps so much easier and more pleasant. Look at how men act at the office. Those who eat slow-burning carbos give up the nervous energy of the sugar junkie for quiet calm and lots of powerful energy in reserve. They stand at the ready for crisis with a surplus of energy for the more mundane chores of daily living. The sugar junkie is living from one food-created crisis to another. When a real crisis erupts, he's hot-tempered and out of steam.

Chapter 6

Get Hard

MONDAY THROUGH FRIDAY, DURING JANUARY 1992, I LEFT THE SET OF *CBS* *This Morning* for the World Gym at 7:45 A.M. I'd take with me the newspapers and that day's medical journals. At the gym I'd climb onto an Alpine Climber. This is a huge mega-stairclimber with steps three times as long as the average StairMaster. It also has a nicely laid out series of bars on which to lay my papers and journals so I can work while working out. But toward the end of each successive week, I'd have to drag myself in the front door of the gym. Almost imperceptibly, over the course of ninety minutes on the Alpine Climber, I'd crumble from an upright posture into a bent, lumbering, painful gait. The slower and more crippled I crawled away, I figured, the better my workout. "Go till you drop!" "No pain no gain" echoed in my brain whenever I began to slow.

While researching a piece on the vitamin industry, I came across a copy of Dr. Michael Colgan's *Optimum Sports Nutrition* at a health food store. For any kind of serious athlete it read like an action-packed thriller. I could barely put it down. In example after example I'd say, "Hey that's me! That's me too." Like many endurance athletes, I'd endlessly grazed on pastas, breads, and cereals. I'd ignored adequate amounts of protein and feasted on poor-quality, highly fattening carbos. I'd followed the conventional wisdom that all Americans get excess amounts of protein. Then I added up my total daily protein intake. It was less than 60 percent of the traditional Recommended Daily Allowances! For the amount of exercise I do, the book said, I needed 150 percent of the RDA. I began to eat the right amounts of high-quality protein. I experienced one of those stunning, black-and-white, overnight, "Hey-this-really-works" kind of differences. My back and leg pain went away. During weight-training workouts, I began to make huge gains for the first time in my life. Instead of aimlessly grazing on carbos day and night, I concentrated my carbohydrates around my workouts to fuel and refuel. I just couldn't believe it. Here I had thought old age had grabbed me by the ankles and pulled me down for one last gasp. Suddenly I had all the energy I needed. Every workout was strong. The gains in strength and muscle mass were tremendous. Like most responsible physicians, I had been taken in by the nutritional establishment and led to believe that three squares from the basic food groups were all I really needed. What a mistake! After polling dozens of my friends with my newfound insight, I came to realize that they too could barely crawl through a workout because they just didn't have the onboard fuel or protein to give themselves a chance.

The conventional wisdom is that most Americans get too much protein. Read most books on nutrition and that's what you'll be told. If you're fatigued, prone to frequent infections, make little progress with your workouts, or are just too tired to exercise, consider too little protein as a possible cause. Dr. Michael Colgan, the director of the Colgan Institute, a nutritional analysis group in San Diego, says, "Uninformed physicians, nutritionists, and dieticians (often funded by the meat or dairy industry) parrot the RDA as right for everyone."

Conventional Wisdom:
Don't worry about protein, you get more than enough.
New Paradigm:
Protein's a real problem. You can't get strong, lean, high-quality muscle without the right amount of high-quality protein.

The Image

Paint a vivid image of weak, shriveled, old muscles draped over thinning bone. See your posture hunched forward, your gait marred by a slight stoop. Now visualize crystalline pure amino acids coursing through your bloodstream into your muscles. Every time you work those muscles, picture how they are bathed in powerful nutrients. Daily, those muscles harden and grow. Your shoulders are thrown back, your waistline narrows, and fat is stripped from your frame.

WHERE MEN GO WRONG

Pasta Junkies: Just Not Enough

The popularity of carbohydrate loading among athletes prompted many Americans to adopt a high-carbohydrate diet. The National Cancer Institute, American Heart Association, and others promote the idea of eating more carbos. That, however, is often misinterpreted to mean nearly all carbos, to the exclusion of protein. I'll be the first to admit that I've existed on pasta lunches and dinners for years, but eating pastas, grains, breads, and bagels can leave you seriously deficient in muscle-building protein. A whole generation of runners have starved themselves of protein, and many look it. They are thin to a fault, stripped of upper-body muscle, and walk with a bent, hobbled gait. Dr. Bill Evans, the director of the Noll Physiological Research Center at Pennsylvania State University, has demonstrated that endurance athletes may need more protein than the current RDA. Since protein is used during continuous aerobic exercise, and since the body does not store protein as a fuel, you can theoretically begin chewing up muscle to use as a source of protein. During aerobic exercise, 5 to 10 percent of calories burned are protein, but if your muscle runs out of carbohydrate, up to 15 percent of the calories consumed come from proteins.

The syndrome of too much carbohydrate and not enough protein is most graphically demonstrated in Southeast Asia. Rice paddy workers have notably thin bodies with little fat and little muscle. The reason is simple: they eat lots of high-quality carbohydrates, which keeps their fat down, but they have a very low intake of protein, so they never develop any muscle mass. When these same people emigrate to the United States, many are transformed into muscular individuals as a result of a higher-protein diet.

No Gainer: Pumping Iron Without the Iron

Scientific studies have demonstrated that you need more protein than the RDA specifies to build new muscle. Beginning bodybuilders require more than experienced bodybuilders but are less likely to get it.

Nouveau Vegetarian: Too Little of the Right Kind

There is a widespread trend toward a pseudo-vegetarian diet, which sharply cuts down on animal and dairy protein sources. However, the pseudo-vegetarian is not well versed in how to be a vegetarian, so he falls far short of his protein goals. Only by mixing and matching the right foods can you get complete proteins that build and maintain muscle. But in a half-hearted or ill-thought-through effort to be vegetarian, many of us fall flat on our faces. If you eat a mostly vegetarian diet, you need to know how to do it. The core concept is that you must complement grains with beans, beans with grains, or either with a complete protein. You also need to increase your intake of foods that contain iron, zinc, and B vitamins, which you might not otherwise get with a makeshift vegetarian diet.

Too Much Protein: Powder Mania

Walk into any health food store and you'll find a section with huge tubs of protein powder with extremely muscular-looking men on the labels. Serious bodybuilders can roll through several hundred grams of protein a day. At a certain point, this can become dangerous. Bodybuilders complain of bone pain and kidney pain when they overload. Too much protein can wash out calcium and thin your bones, which is more of a problem for women than men. Large excesses of protein can overload your kidneys and result in high levels of blood urea nitrogen.

There's the charge that excess protein may cause cancer, although there are no convincing studies. Part of the cancer risk may come from proteins that come with lots of excess fat or are seared or blackened during cooking. How much is too much? At levels five times the RDA you're headed for real trouble with no promise of any benefit. Two and a half times the RDA is the maximum safe limit and that's only for a professional athlete who trains or competes vigorously three hours or more a day.

Too Little Protein: Dieters' Dilemma

Popular weight-loss programs strip protein from your muscles as fast as they strip fat. In fact, only 40 percent of weight loss from a calorie-restricted diet may be fat. That's why you should be consuming at least 125 percent of your RDA for protein if you're on an old-fashioned, calorie-restricted diet.

Too Much of the Wrong Protein: Steak and Burgers

If you eat a traditional meat-and-potatoes diet or eat at fast-food hamburger outlets, you're probably getting all the protein you need. What you're getting with that protein is far more saturated fat than is good for you. Without modern nutrition it simply wouldn't be possible to have lean, muscular athletes. Look at two American heroes at two ends of this century: Teddy Roosevelt and Arnold Schwarzenegger. Teddy was a big guy, but clearly carried a hefty amount of body fat. Arnold's also a big guy, but carries almost no body fat. The difference is the kind of protein these two men ate. Packing on lots of extra fat calories with your protein serves no performance purpose and is an independent risk factor for heart disease. Doctors worry, too, about the problem of iron overload and its risks of cancer and heart disease, since some Americans have a tendency to store too much iron with heavy red-meat diets.

Chronic Fatigue

Cliff Sheats, a controversial Dallas-based nutritionist, finds that hundreds of his customers come to him complaining of fatigue. These men do not necessarily have the official "chronic fatigue syndrome," but they complain of unending, bone-gnawing fatigue. No treatment appears to improve them. A nutritional analysis shows two findings: first, Sheats says, a crash-and-burn diet that wears them out (as described in Chapter 5); second, these men eat too few calories and even less protein. By increasing the amount of protein and increasing calories in general, many of them no longer have the symptoms of chronic fatigue.

WHAT REALLY WORKS

Step One

Assess your level of activity to determine your protein needs.

Level 1: You are sedentary and don't plan to change.

Level 2: You are a seasoned bodybuilder who trains four days a week.

Level 3: You are a serious aerobic athlete training sixty to ninety minutes a day.

Level 4: You are just beginning a program of building substantial amounts of young muscle and plan to train at least four days a week.

Level 5: Practically speaking, this is the upper limit sports scientists are willing to recommend and only if you train or compete more than three hours a day in punishing events such as the Tour de France. Dr. Peter Lemon of Kent State University in Kent, Ohio, has done research that demonstrates that athletes with normal kidney function can handle slightly more protein without any bad effects but also without any apparent benefit.

Keep in mind that these are simply suggested levels. Although researchers I interviewed have good studies to support these levels, they don't like to prescribe specific amounts of protein until this young field can provide more answers about safety and effectiveness. Keep a diary to see if these levels work for you. If you are concerned about safety, have your doctor draw a test for blood urea nitrogen to ascertain if you are overloading. If this sounds dangerous, keep in mind that the average American on a red-meat-and-potatoes diet eats the amount of protein suggested for level four. On days you don't train, you don't need the extra protein.

Step Two

Now find your activity level across the top of the chart on the next page. Follow down that column until you find your weight in pounds. That's the maximum grams of protein intake per day for which there is any scientific support.

Here are the values by which the chart was calculated in grams of protein per pound of body weight.

1. 0.36 gm/lb = current RDA
2. 0.55 gm/lb = trained bodybuilder
3. 0.59 gm/lb = endurance athlete
4. 0.77 gm/lb = novice bodybuilder
5. 0.91 gm/lb = practical safe upper limit

Step Three

Plan for your protein intake. Since there is no storage form of protein, you can use only so much at a sitting. Experts put that at 30 to 40 grams. I plan my daily eating around my protein intake, then I add carbohydrates. I like to get a protein hit first thing in the morning before I exercise. The protein wakes me up like caffeine but without the buzz and crash. Right after exercise is the best opportunity, since it can best build new muscle at that time. I like to get some protein with midmorning and midafternoon snacks as well as lunch to stay sharp. Carbohydrate meals without protein make most men drowsy. Since too much protein in the evening makes it hard to fall asleep, I eat less protein and more carbos for dinner. Protein is also a terrific satiator, so you'll feel less hungry eating protein than any other food. By including protein in all your meals and snacks, you'll cut down on the amount you eat. I've always eaten a big breakfast, at least 700 calories. I was still ravenously hungry by noon

	Level of Activity				
	1	2	3	4	5
Weight					
100	36	55	59	77	91
110	40	60	65	85	100
120	44	65	71	93	109
130	47	71	77	100	118
140	51	76	83	108	127
150	55	82	89	116	136
160	58	87	95	124	145
170	62	93	100	131	155
180	65	98	106	139	164
190	69	104	112	147	173
200	73	109	118	155	182
210	76	115	124	162	191
220	80	120	130	170	200
230	84	125	136	178	209
240	87	131	142	185	218
250	91	136	148	193	227
260	95	142	154	201	236

and could pack away another 1,000 calories. By increasing my morning protein, I almost have to force myself to eat at lunch.

If you're too busy or harried to get all your protein in real foods, you could consider supplements. Some of these are a real rip-off. They just don't have the quality or quantity of protein they claim. Others are highly controversial because they add a kitchen sink worth of stimulants, energizers, and growth factors. I'll put it on the record, though, that I take these supplements and believe there is a real role for them, as long as you're getting most of your protein from foods. Some people just can't eat the extra meal or calories to get the extra protein. There's also an argument that protein should be taken before, during, and after workouts. As a supplement, it's easier to get into your system at those times than real food. See Chapter 11 for the real dirt. I usually drink 40 grams of protein right after my workout.

Protein needs carbohydrate to make its way into muscle. Animal protein does bump up your insulin slightly but not enough to transport the individual amino acids into your muscle. Dr. Richard Wurtman of MIT says that you need about 200 calories of carbohydrate to nurse along the protein you've eaten. That's enough to increase your insulin levels to increase the transport of amino acids into your muscle.

Step Four

Eat quality protein. Just as important as getting high-quality protein is getting high quality without too much excess baggage. I've included two separate tables on the following pages. The first rates protein quality from highest to lowest quality. The second rates protein by the amount of fat that comes with it. You'll observe that the highest-quality proteins can also be the leanest.

Highest-Quality Protein Food Sources (based on the protein efficiency ratio)

Here's how proteins are rated for their ability to build muscle. High-quality proteins are a real advantage because you may get away with less if you're trying to watch your calories.

Whey
Whole egg
Egg whites
Casein–milk protein
Skim milk
Milk and cheese
Fish
Lean meat and chicken
Maize
Rice
Wheat
Oatmeal
Peanut butter
Soy flour

Table provided by American Dietetic Association nutritionist Alicia Moag-Stahlberg, M.S., R.D.

Lean Proteins

This table shows how much fat you get with your protein. The number to key in on is "protein as a % of calories." Leading the list of proteins high in quality protein and low in fat is egg protein powder at 96 percent. At the low end is a fast-food hamburger with only 17 percent of calories as protein. Choose your proteins so they don't contain too much excess fat.

Food	Amount	Calories	Protein (grams)	Protein as a % of calories	Fat (grams)
Protein powder, egg	2 hpg tbsp	100	24	96	0
Protein powder, milk and egg	2 hpg tbsp	110	25	91	0
Protein powder, soy	2 hpg tbsp	80	18	90	0
Egg white (chicken)	1 large	16	3.4	85	0
Egg, whole (chicken)	1 large	79	6.1	31	5.6
Yeast, dry, baker's	1 oz	80	10.5	52	0.5
Chicken breast without skin, roasted	½ breast/ 3 oz	142	26.7	75	3.1
Turkey breast without skin, roasted	3.5 oz	157	29.9	76	3.2
Fish, cod, baked	3 oz	89	19.4	87	0.7
Fish, tuna, white, canned in water	3 oz	116	22.7	78	2.1

Food	Amount	Calories	Protein (grams)	Protein as a % of calories	Fat (grams)
Fish, flounder, baked	3.5 oz	202	30	59	8.2
Fish, salmon, canned	3 oz	130	17.4	54	6.2
Pork tenderloin, trimmed, roasted	3.5 oz	166	28.8	69	4.8
Venison, lean, raw	3 oz	107	17.9	67	3.4
Round steak, trimmed, broiled	3.5 oz	191	31.7	66	6.2
Ground beef, extra lean, baked	3.5 oz	274	30.3	44	16
Cottage cheese, dry curd	1 cup	123	25	81	0.6
Cottage cheese, 2% fat	1 cup	203	31.1	61	4.4
American cheese	2 oz (slices)	212	12.6	24	17.8
Peanut butter, smooth	2 tbsp	188	9	19	16
Kidney beans, boiled	1 cup	225	15.4	27	0.9
Big Mac hamburger (McDonald's)	1 burger	570	24.6	17	35

Table provided by Dr. Luke Bucci of SpectraCell Labs.

Chapter 7

Eat All You Want

YOU STAND TALL AND FIRM, YOUR CAREFULLY BENCH-PRESSED CHEST thrust forward. Dressed in an oversized surfing T-shirt and baggy surfing shorts, you're the model of a male in his prime. As you wait for the elevator to take you down to your racing bike, an attractive female colleague comes forward, places her hand on your stomach, and then gently presses a roll of fat between her thumb and forefinger. They do not meet. Separating them by an inch or more is a roll of fat. How unattractive, her eyes say. You try to protest but firmly resolve then and there to get rid of that roll once and for all. Later that evening you reassess. You've already cut down on the fat in your diet. You exercise. How's it going to come off? A diet!

You're a tough guy. Breakfast time goes by without a single calorie. By midmorning, your brain can barely focus on your desktop, your blood sugar has fallen through the floor. By noon, daggerlike pangs of hunger. Your speaking voice is hollow. You don't have the mental energy to do more than crawl through an important afternoon presentation. You reach under your shirt to squeeze the roll around your waist. It's smaller! Motivation to continue. You're tough all right, but going quicker than the fat is hard-won lean muscle.

The sacrifice of that muscle represents the loss of vitality, energy, and youth.

Conventional Wisdom:
Eat less to weigh less.
New Paradigm:
Eat all you want.

After Europeans return home from visiting American theme parks, what are they most apt to tell their friends about?

a. Epcot
b. The Magic Kingdom
c. Jurassic Park
d. MGM Grand
e. The balloon people

The answer is (e) the balloon people. Unknown in most of the world, balloon people don't look as if they're meant to be fat. However, so much fat is unmistakably present that it appears to be popping out of their skin, giving them an unnatural balloonlike appearance. Balloon people are seen wobbling from one food stand to another, grazing on soft drinks, french fries, and cheeseburgers at America's theme parks, malls, movie complexes, and fast-food outlets. The balloon people represent the extreme of the undue influence modern foods can have over our willpower and decision-making skills.

Balloon people, through little fault of their own, are lured into eating foods that evade elaborate and sensitive brain controls that regulate the amount of body fat we're supposed to have. Meat and potatoes drenched with fat, processed foods stuffed with stripped sugars, and fattened baked goods outsmart all the brain's sophisticated protective abilities to control weight. Balloon people are cued by smells, suggestive food ads, and a privileged sense of the right to eat. Psychologists would describe them as little better than lab rats, trapped in an environment from which they cannot escape. To Europeans, they look like herds of animals who aimlessly graze from one food source to another throughout the day.

The irony is that these people could eat masses of food and lose weight. Any one of these people could shed body fat, rid himself of hunger, slash his risk of disease, and create boundless energy by simply changing foods, even without exercise. Sadly, most balloon people make the wrong choice when they want to pop the balloon.

I want to make a very sharp distinction between the balloon people, whose weight is propped up by massive amounts of terrible foods, and those who are genetically obese, whom I by no means wish to insult. Most have applied tremendous resolve and hard work to lose weight but are hampered by their own biology. I do not mean to trivialize the extreme difficulty they have in losing weight and keeping it off.

Dieting has no real place in weight loss. A recent survey by *Consumer Reports* reinforced what weight researchers have said for years: diets just don't work. The failure rate of dieting equals the failure rate of treating lung cancer! That's about 95 percent. Dieting destroys your ability to lose and keep weight off by lowering your metabolic rate. Instead of running like a finely tuned engine on high, burning fat even as you rest, metabolism drops to a rate not much faster than that of a hibernating grizzly. Dieting also destroys many pounds of active muscle that could work hard to keep you lean. That loss of muscle mass is like aging ten years in six weeks.

Big Eddie was a native Hawaiian who weighed in at 425 pounds and lived on the island of Oahu. His blood sugar rose as high as 800, his cholesterol was nearly 400. He required 60 units of insulin a day, and emptied four full Hefty garbage bags full of medications each year. Eddie's diet was packed with fats, processed foods, and sugars. His doctor, Terry Shintani, asked Eddie to return to the foods of his ancestors. He sold Eddie on the strong spiritual values of the foods his forefathers thrived on, a diet that was rich in native fruits and vegetables. He was allowed to eat all he wanted as long as he stayed native. Dr. Shintani showed Eddie pictures of nineteenth-century Hawaiians: tall, strong, and lean. In several months Eddie's weight plummeted. His blood sugar dropped. His cholesterol fell into a normal range. He no longer required insulin. He no longer spent his days taking dozens of medications. He lost 150 pounds by eating more food, lots more food! The usual weight-loss strategies had completely failed Big Eddie. Only by shifting to a new paradigm did he lose big time. His new bearings were clear:

- Eat the spiritual food of your ancestors.
- Eat all you want to lose weight.

What happened? Native Hawaiian foods are rich in nutrients but sparse in fat and processed and simple sugars. Even if he gorged himself, he couldn't eat more than a couple of thousand calories a day without calorie-dense foods. The lack of fats and the control of his blood sugar level deprived his body of its most efficient ways of storing excess fat. African Americans could also benefit enormously by eating the spiritual and cultural food of their ancestors in African countries where foods are high in complex carbohydrates and low in fats. Experts believe that their high rate of diabetes, high cholesterol, obesity, and high blood pressure could be reduced substantially by choosing from many of the spectacular sub-Saharan African diets.

The notion of eating more to lose fat is so foreign to most Americans that it inspires a pathological fear. My first trip as a team physician for the U.S. Ski Team was to Grand Targee. I was stunned by the amount of food the men on the team ate. The women, on the other hand, ate nearly nothing. They figured that lots of early-season exercise combined with the use of a low-calorie diet would help them lose that summer fat. Wrong! These kids nearly died. They had no energy, couldn't race, and were almost sent home. What was wrong? They needed to prime the pump to lose weight by eating more of the right foods.

Consider two men in their eighties. Who would you rather become? A thin, wiry, skeletal figure with ashen color and wax-museum-quality translucent skin? Or a robust figure with a lifeguard's physique, ruddy complexion, and ear-to-ear grin? They represent two strikingly different theories of eating and aging. The first eighty-year-old eats little food, less than 1,500 calories per day. The other figure is represented by Walt Stack, who was at the age of eighty-four a senior triathlete who packed in over 4,000 calories a day. What's the difference? The first man represents a leading theory of aging that advocates a lifelong low-calorie diet as the best way to grow very old. That's based on lab rat data and the observation that some societies with very long-lived elders eat very little food. There's no proof that a low-calorie diet actually works to extend life in humans. There's no room for error in this kind of diet. With so few calories, each one must count and deliver a wallop of protein, carbohydrate, minerals and vitamins. These small eaters are ascetic, monklike figures whose metabolism turns over so slowly that researchers believe they may save enough wear and tear on their body's metabolism to eke out a few more years of existence. But what if you follow in their footsteps and the scientists are wrong? You've suffered a life of restraint and misery for nothing!

Is there another choice besides slowing your metabolism down to a crawl? Sure! Crank up your metabolism. Walt's body worked like a huge furnace burning at full tilt. He ate plenty of food, maintained lots of lean muscle, and remained very active. Keeping big healthy muscles brimming with food-based energy stores kept his metabolism revved up like that of a twenty-year-old.

WHAT REALLY WORKS

Turn Down the Density, Increase the Volume

Big Eddie lost 150 pounds by increasing the amount he ate, but decreasing the calorie density of the foods he ate. By eating dense foods like hamburgers, fries, candy bars, and soft drinks, he could pack 4,000 calories into his stomach. But Big Eddie could pack his stomach to the bursting point with native Hawaiian low-density foods and barely get 800 calories in. Since so many of those low-density calories were slow-burning carbos, he wasn't hungry for hours afterward. He simply couldn't pile in enough food in a day to keep his weight at 425. High-density foods are fats, sugars, and processed foods. Cliff Sheats, author of *Lean Bodies,* finds that many men are "fat virgins" but still can't lose weight. By fat virgins he means that they've already cut most of the fat from their diet. Where do they go wrong? They eat lots of processed foods and white-flour-based bagels, pastas, breads, cereals, muffins, and crackers.

Eat Foods When You Need Them

Americans have a curious tradition of eating the most food when it will do us the least good and the most harm. Dinner has become the centerpiece of most Americans' nutritional lives, but dinner is as close as you can come to mainlining food. The inactivity after dinner followed by a full night's sleep opens an enormous gateway for fat to line our coronary arteries and pack on extra pounds of body fat. Food has its biggest benefit at breakfast. It wakes up the body and increases metabolism. An active morning burns many of those calories. When does food do the most good? When taken to fuel activity and exercise. It's at this time that you can remove guilt and enjoy your food. Food eaten in the hours before a workout is burned up during and after a workout because of the increase in body metabolism. Food eaten immediately after a workout helps to refuel muscles and will also be burned at a faster rate because metabolism remains elevated for so long after exercise. So if you pack most of your calories into breakfast and surrounding your workout, you can enjoy more food with less worry about gaining weight. Try going to bed hungry. You'll sleep better and shed extra pounds of fat with ease.

Don't Be Afraid to Let Go

The tenet held most firmly by anyone trying to lose weight is that you have to eat less food. Nutrition's biggest paradigm shift ever is that you should eat more to lose body fat. That has been the theme of several popular books, including *Lean Bodies* by Cliff Sheats and *Eat More, Weigh Less* by Dr. Dean Ornish.

Eat Thermogenic Foods

Ever lie awake at night after a big steak dinner as your heart goes boom boom boom so hard your chest wall bounces while your stomach pitches and rolls? Well, that's the metabolic effect of food on your digestive system. Simply put, your stomach and intestine are going full tilt to digest your dinner. Hard to get to sleep? You bet. Why? Your digestive system is doing the equivalent of an eight-minute mile while you try to sleep. You're feeling the thermic effects of food. The higher a food's thermic effect, the more energy your body must expend in order to digest it.

Fat has very little thermic effect, because it doesn't take much energy to digest fat. Protein and carbohydrates take a lot more energy to digest.

The thermic effect is determined by a food's effect on the following:

- The stomach's emptying rate.
- Its breakup into food components in the intestine.
- Its absorption into the bloodstream.
- Its effect on hormones like insulin.

Eat high-thermic foods like proteins and whole grains during the morning and afternoon but avoid them in large quantities during the hours before bedtime so they don't prevent you from sleeping.

Eat Slow-Burning Carbos

There are big differences in how fast carbohydrates break down. The slower they break down, the more energy your body expends, and the fewer calories will end up around your belly. For example, a tablespoon of sugar takes a lot less energy to digest than a thick slice of coarse European bread.

The Glycemic Index accurately reflects which carbohydrates are and which aren't metabolically active. A food high on the Glycemic Index, like white bread, takes minimal effort to digest. If it's low on the Glycemic Index, like lentils, it generates lots of metabolic activity to extract the carbohydrate from fiber and other food components. Digesting it or moving it around or breaking it down all take more effort.

The most important factor determining the thermic effect of foods is when you eat them. Breakfast has a thermic effect, because it increases your metabolism. In essence, part of the calories you eat during breakfast you get for free! If you eat foods or drink supplements before you exercise, a hunk of those calories won't count either. They'll be chewed up both by exercise itself and the higher metabolic rate that follows for hours afterward. So eat a good breakfast, because it cranks up your metabolism, makes you feel energetic, and allows you to eat some free calories. Taken properly before exercise, a good meal contains lots of free calories and vastly improves the quality of your workout and how you feel during your workout. However, since lots of food in your stomach during exercise can be very unpleasant, you need to plan what you will eat and how long before exercise to get the best result.

Beware of Too Much Fructose

Fructose may pose a real problem for anyone trying to control his weight. Top bodybuilders avoid too much fructose because it can go to fat around the belly. Large quantities of fructose go directly to the liver, where they can be turned into a fat called a triglyceride. In about a third of Americans, fructose can also increase blood cholesterol. Dr. Judith Hallfrisch of the USDA says, "We've given 7.5 percent to 15 percent of calories of added fructose, instead of complex carbohydrates, and gotten increases in total cholesterol, LDL, and triglycerides. Even people with normal insulin responses had an increase in triglycerides. In my opinion we consume levels of sugars that are high enough to cause these effects."

So if you're trying to control your weight by eating fewer simple sugars or watching your blood-fat levels, beware of too much fructose. This fat-boosting action of fructose is a real concern because of the rapidly increasing use of high-fructose corn sweetener in soft drinks and other processed foods. I don't avoid fructose altogether, but I'd rather have superslow carbos. While it's widely assumed that orange, grapefruit, and other fruit juices are good for you, processed juices are deficient in most naturally occurring minerals and vitamins. There is a slogan in the health food community: "Processed juices [such as orange juice] are to fruit what white flour is to whole grain."

Many are heavily fortified, but that doesn't make the underlying beverage anything terrific. The main naturally occurring sugar in fruit juices is fructose. Better to eat the fruit.

Count Your Fat

Dr. Dean Ornish and Pritikin advocate diets with as little as 10 percent fat. Since a calorie of fat can put twice as much fat on your body as a calorie of carbohydrate, substantial weight loss occurs by simply substituting slow-burning carbos for fat calories. In fact, a man in China eating the same number of calories and performing the same level of activity as a man of similar stature in America will weigh up to twenty pounds less just because he eats carbos instead of fat. To stay in the range of a 10 percent fat diet, many nutritionists advocate counting grams of fat. With the FDA's new food labels, your job is a lot simpler than it used to be. Any of a number of fat counting books can help you keep track of the fat found in meats, fast foods, and restaurant foods. Here's how many grams of fat you can eat at each calorie level for a 10 percent fat diet (Pritikin, Ornish) and for a 20 percent (American Heart Association) low-fat diet.

Calories	10% fat	20% fat
1,000	11 g	22 g
1,500	17 g	33 g
2,000	22 g	44 g
2,500	28 g	56 g
3,000	33 g	67 g
3,500	39 g	78 g
4,000	44 g	89 g
4,500	50 g	100 g

My personal belief is that it is far easier to just eat the low-fat foods you'll read about in the following chapters than it is to count fat grams. However, if you're going to stick with standard American fare, counting grams of fat is a must.

To some people it seems looney to give up fruit juices, pastas, bagels, white bread, and other processed foods. However, as a strategy to lower your body fat, it's much better than the alternative, which is eating like a bird. Rather than focusing on what you can't eat, let's look at the vast universe of terrific foods you can choose that will allow you to eat what you want and still lose fat.

Chapter 8

Multicultural Eating

IF EATING HAS BECOME THE KIND OF CHORE THAT'S MADE MUCH OF LIFE in late-twentieth-century America little fun, try multicultural eating. Rather than fussing and picking from an à la carte menu of increasingly meager choices, treat yourself to a whole new world of eating. Most of us are creatures of habit when it comes to food. President Clinton loves his french fries; the caricatured American male has steak and potatoes for dinner every evening. Sure, our diet is more varied than that, but surveys show that we still have basic meals we stick to. I have the same breakfast and lunch almost every day. William Castelli, M.D., director of the Framingham Heart Study in Massachusetts, put the problem to me this way: "Most people have ten favorite nutritionally terrible meals that they recycle over and over year in and year out. If they'd just pick ten new meals and fall into the habit of eating them, they could accomplish all their nutritional goals."

Okay, so what are the ten new meals? A variety of cultures eat remarkably healthy diets right across the board. If you eat within certain cultures, you don't need to worry about counting calories, counting grams of fat, or measuring portion sizes. Just pick up the menu, order, and eat. Learning to shop for and cook ethnic foods quickly becomes a matter of habit. Use the information in this chapter to make your first several choices more discerning than usual. Once you've hit upon your ten new meals, ordering or cooking them will become second nature.

Conventional Wisdom:

Good nutrition means giving up everything you ever enjoyed about eating. Learn to eat sprouts and like it.

New Paradigm:

Eating is a fascinating, life-long adventure.

Don't learn how to eat bad food well; learn to eat great new foods instead. Invest in your health and your youth by eating foods that cultures have spent thousands of years refining and honing into great-tasting, satisfying meals.

What Multicultural Eating Will Do for You

1. Increase slow-burning carbos.
2. Decrease all fats.
3. Decrease all simple sugars.
4. Increase fiber.

Good cooks have little trouble making healthy foods taste terrific, but most of us aren't gourmet chefs who can experiment with different combinations of basic ingredients. That's why venturing into different cultures is the simplest way to eat really well. I know from my own experimentation in the kitchen that I do poorly trying to turn supernutritious foods into anything better than sawdust soup. That's why multicultural nutrition is such a terrific shortcut.

Traditional healthy cultures have learned how to make foods delicious without simply dumping in fat and sugar. Scientists have discovered that exceptionally healthy diets are inexpensive, unprocessed fare, precisely the kind that people abandon once they become affluent. People of the ancient world had been eating light, healthy diets long before scientists discovered they were the world's most therapeutic cuisines.

You may find your commitment to multicultural eating strengthened by an understanding of the food's history, symbolism, or healing values. In Okinawa, for example, more people live to age one hundred than any other place on earth. Okinawans trust in the magic of food to give them long life. Foods packed with vital nutrients keep them strong decades longer than most of us could ever hope to live. If your family is descended from a culture that practices terrific nutrition, you may find it easier to sell yourself and your family on eating within your own culture by embracing the spiritual and cultural values of its food. If you come from a nutritionally disastrous culture, adopt a culture for its youth-building, life-saving foods. New research is proving that multicultural eating has strong healing properties. When heart attack victims were placed on a Mediterranean diet, 17 percent fewer patients died than those on the American Heart Association's Heart Savers Diet. These heart patients delighted in the license to drink red wine and eat dazzling Italian foods instead of suffering on a restricted, heart-healthy diet.

Multicultural eating means freedom from most of the worry about the mistakes made in trying to eat well. There are, to be sure, pitfalls. In each of the following sections I'll point out where you can go astray. Americans have a way of perverting good foods. True Mexican foods are enormously healthful, but served in American restaurants, they become killer burritos, heartburn enchiladas, and fat-to-the-belly tacos. Why? To suit the American palate, many Mexican restaurants in the United States add lard-based beans, sour cream, white-flour burritos, and buttered rice. I order a chicken burrito for lunch several days a week from a local shop called California Burrito. It comes with enough sour cream, guacamole, and jack cheese to make a fast-food aficionado blush. I order it without those three items and find the burrito still tastes really terrific. But ethnic restaurants fear offending Americans by not giving them enough fat. While the Chinese eat a great diet in China, dishes like mu shu pork served in America contain twice the cholesterol of a McDonald's Egg McMuffin.

Throughout this chapter you will find suggestions about butter or cream or other add-ons you can ask to have removed from a dish. Wahida Karmally, M.S., R.D., director of nutrition at the Irving Center for Clinical Research, at Columbia Presbyterian Medical Center in New York, says that fear of lawsuits makes restaurants quite attentive to people with food allergies, but "they really don't care if you have a high cholesterol level." So a good trick is to say that you are allergic to anything that you really don't want in your dish.

MEDITERRANEAN

When forty-three-year-old Maurilio DeZolt beat dozens of kids half his age to win a gold medal in the Lillehammer cross-country relay race, where did he place the credit for his victory? "The Mediterranean diet. Pasta, red wine, and olive oil." Nutritionists, research scientists, and epidemiologists affiliated with Oldways Preservation & Exchange Trust in Boston agree. They've discovered that the people living in and around the Mediterranean in 1960 had the lowest rates of chronic disease in the world and a life expectancy among the highest.

The principle of the traditional Mediterranean diet of 1960 is that foods from plant sources form the core of the diet, while foods from animal sources form the fringe. Men drink one or two glasses of wine a day, primarily with meals. Research suggests that it is unlikely that the Mediterranean diet would be as protective against chronic diseases if moderate wine consumption were eliminated from the diet. Oldways recommends that Americans consider wine consumption, unless consumption would put the individual or others at risk.

Olive oil is the region's traditional fat. Olive oil, which is high in monounsaturated fatty acids, lowers the "bad cholesterol" (known as LDL), whereas butter, beef fat, other fats from land animals, and partially hydrogenated fats commonly consumed in margarines can increase bad cholesterol. Olive oil also contains substantial amounts of antioxidants, which may prevent bad cholesterol deposits from forming and blocking arteries. If you want to follow the Mediterranean diet, olive oil should replace and not be added to other fats. Fresh, minimally processed foods may explain the protective levels of antioxidants and other micronutrients in their diets.

Traditional southern Italian cuisine heads the pack of healthy and delicious Mediterranean diets. But beware of contemporary northern Italian cooking! The north uses more butter and dairy products as well as meat. The south uses little meat, olive oil, and more beans, fruits, and vegetables. Compared with northern Italians of the same economic class, southern Italians consume one-third less beef and veal and four-fifths less butter. Southern Italians eat one-fifth more bread, pasta, vegetables, and fruit and twice as much fish.

What to Eat

Contrary to the popular perception of Italian food as all pasta and pizza, fresh vegetables — from broccoli, eggplant, tomatoes, leafy greens, mushrooms, potatoes, fennel, lima and fava beans to zucchini — are at the heart of the ideal southern Italian diet. The pasta is nearly fat free and eaten as an appetizer, while seafood, chicken, or shellfish is the main course. For dessert, fresh fruit is served. Although people in Mediterranean cultures eat at least three times as much bread as Americans, it is rarely buttered. I would modify the Mediterranean diet by purchasing whole-grain pastas and breads, as recommended in Chapter 5, "Control Your Blood Sugar."

What to Avoid

Ohio State University professor Gordon Wardlaw says that Americanized chefs add heavy cheese, meat, cream-based sauces, and fatty or deep-fried meat and fish to the Italian menu. Say no to that extra Parmesan cheese. Even a single tablespoon adds two grams of fat, of which one is saturated. Watch out for cannelloni, ravioli, lasagna, and tortellini. They're usually stuffed with heavy cheeses and fatty meats. Other dishes to avoid include:

- Meat and cheese antipasto.
- Fried mixed seafood or meat called fritto misto.

- Fried calamari, which has more cholesterol than a four-egg omelet.

Also, beware of pastas with rich cream sauces, such as Alfredo and carbonara (bacon and egg yolks in a cream sauce). According to the Center for Science in the Public Interest (CSPI), a nonprofit health-advocacy organization in Washington, D.C., fettuccini Alfredo has as much saturated fat as three pints of Breyers Butter Almond Ice Cream. Avoid adding pepperoni or sausage to pizza. Avoid smoked pork (capiccola) and fatty ham like prosciutto.

CSPI conducted an investigation of Italian food sold in the United States. Its opinion of Italian dishes found in American restaurants: You can find low-fat entrees. "An order of spaghetti or linguine with any sauce on top, except cream sauce or pesto, is going to make the grade," but "Most entrees supply at least 1,500 mg. of sodium, making it tough to stay under your 1,800 to 2,400 mg. daily limit." CSPI also says that vegetables are pretty scarce. Here's how CSPI would make it better:

- Instead of garlic bread, eat plain Italian bread — no butter.
- Make spaghetti with meatballs better by asking for meatballs in a tomato sauce instead of a fattier meat sauce.
- Make chicken marsala better by asking for a lot less sauce.
- Make spaghetti with sausage better by ordering the sausage in tomato sauce.
- Order certain meals without the cheese topping. If you do so with veal parmigiana, you'll cut a quarter of the fat; with eggplant parmigiana, you'll save yourself from eating almost two-thirds the fat; with cheese manicotti, you won't be eating a quarter of the fat.

Opposite is CSPI's review of the most popular Italian dishes. Pay particular attention to the grams of fat each dish contains.

JAPANESE

The Japanese believe in a harmony between body, community, and nature, which is reflected in their cooking.

Italian dishes	Amount of Dish	Calories	Fat	Cholesterol (mg)	Sodium (mg)
Appetizers					
Spaghetti with tomato sauce	1.5 cups	409	8	14	697
Garlic bread	8 oz	822	40	38	1,083
Fried calamari	3 cups	1,037	70	924	651
Antipasto	1.5 lbs	629	47	131	2,961
Entrees					
Spaghetti with tomato sauce	3.5 cups	849	17	29	1,449
Linguine with red clam sauce	3 cups	892	23	64	2,182
Spaghetti with meat sauce	3 cups	918	25	108	1,792
Linguine with white clam sauce	3 cups	907	29	110	1,881
Spaghetti with meatballs	3.5 cups	1,155	39	163	2,208
*Chicken marsala	10 oz	867	33	175	1,484
Spaghetti with sausage	2.5 cups	1,043	39	114	2,437
*Veal parmigiana	1.5 cups	1,064	44	226	2,043
Cheese ravioli	1.5 cups	623	26	117	1,289
*Eggplant parmigiana	2.5 cups	1,208	62	188	1,999
Cheese manicotti	1.5 cups	695	38	178	1,475
Lasagna	2 cups	968	53	217	2,055
Fettuccini Alfredo	2.5 cups	1,498	97	420	1,029

*Nutritional values for these include 1.5 cups of a side dish of spaghetti with tomato sauce.
Reprinted/adapted from Nutrition Action Healthletter (1875 Connecticut Avenue, N.W., Washington, D.C. 20009-5728).

The traditional staples of the Japanese diet have kept heart disease rates in Japan among the lowest in the civilized world. The introduction of the refrigerator in Japan during the last thirty years has allowed for the use of fresh foods and fewer salted and pickled foods. Refrigerators also allow for more dairy products in the diet. Both changes may be related to the decline in stomach cancer, which has dropped roughly one-third from 1950 to 1982. The benefits of dairy products are supported by a controlled Japanese study showing less stomach cancer in men and women who drink milk daily.

What to Eat

The best carbos are high-quality pure-grain noodles and rice. Protein is found principally in the many soybean products. They are tofu, which is bean curd, soy sauce, and miso, a fermented bean paste.

Popular vegetables are leeks, lettuce, mushrooms, okra, peas, potatoes, pumpkins, sweet potatoes, radishes, rhubarb, seaweed, sorrel, spinach, snow peas, taro, tomatoes, turnips, squash, watercress, and yams. The traditional Japanese eat only small amounts of meat, poultry, and fish. Meat is more a garnish than a main course but still makes up for any amino acids missing from the vegetables and grains. Seaweed, the Japanese lettuce, is chock full of nutrients. Nori, kombu, wakame, hijiki, and a powdered green seaweed called aonoriko are the most common seaweeds used. Oils used are cottonseed, olive, peanut, and sesame seed. The flavoring in Japanese cookery is soy sauce (shoyu), rice wine (sake), vinegar, and sugar. Here are the healthiest dishes to choose:

- "Yakimono," which means broiled. Yakitori is broiled chicken.
- Cucumber salad called sunomono.
- Yosenabe, or fish soup.
- Shabu-shabu is vegetables and meats boiled in broth.
- Chirinabe is a fish stew.
- Sushi and sashimi have become America's favorite healthy import. Be aware that raw fish that hasn't been cleaned properly may contain parasites causing flulike symptoms.
- Dr. Terry Shintani, the director of Preventive Medicine at the Waianae Coast Comprehensive Health Center in Waianae, Hawaii, recommends cold soba noodles (zarusoba) as one of the best Japanese foods to eat as well as vegetable ramen or saimin, vegetable sukiyaki, vegetable sushi with cucumber or yellow pickled turnip, and sushi rice.

The drink at almost every meal is green tea, and fresh fruit is the dessert of choice.

What to Avoid

Salty, smoked, and pickled foods combine to create Japan's two most serious health problems: stroke and stomach cancer. The sodium in salted fish, salty pickled foods, and soy sauce is linked to hypertension and stroke. Go easy on soy or teriyaki sauce to reduce sodium. Salt plus smoked foods rich in nitrates contributes to Japan's elevated rate of stomach cancer, still one of the world's highest. Watch out for tempura, which means batter-dipped and deep-fried. Agemono means deep-fried. Age tofu is fried tofu. Egg dishes such as oyako-donburi and fried pork dishes like tonkatsu are also on the food police's most wanted list.

In the 1950s, fat intake was only 10 to 15 percent of calories consumed in the Japanese diet. It has since doubled. Currently it's about half that of the United States, probably too low to create real heart disease problems. However, fat intake among Japanese teens is equal to that of U.S. teens thanks to fast-food french fries, fried chicken, and burgers. Breast cancer in Japan is on the rise and is thought to be linked to a high fat intake.

MEXICAN

The traditional Mexican diet is built around corn, beans, fish, chicken, and vegetables. The corn is steeped in lime water, adding calcium and free niacin. It's part of every meal and used in tortillas, steamed to make tamales, or served as hot gruel. Beans provide complementary protein so that when corn and beans are eaten together the body can synthesize any protein it needs. Either alone doesn't have enough essential amino acids to meet protein requirements. Mexican food is high in complex carbohydrates and emphasizes the consumption of fruits and vegetables rich in vitamins A and C. Processed foods are not often used, and most dishes are simply prepared and nutritionally balanced. Gordon Wardlaw, associate professor of allied medicine and an expert in human nutrition at Ohio State University, reports that Mexican cuisine "contains lots of fresh vegetables, grilled fish and chicken, and high-fiber, complex carbohydrate beans." Most experts will tell you that Mexican cuisine is healthy and low in fat until it is corrupted by American add-ons. Fatty dishes like beef burritos swimming in melted cheese are not a staple found in Mexico.

What to Eat

Some restaurants allow you to order à la carte tortillas, beans and rice, guacamole, and salsa — diced tomatoes, chilies, and onion. You can make exactly the dish you want at your table. Good choices include:

- Baked tortillas.
- Tomato, onion, and avocado salads with fresh lemon squeezed over the top.
- Shrimp or chicken tostadas on unfried cornmeal tortillas.
- Rice and boiled beans (not refried in lard) are low in fat, high in fiber, and together are complete vegetable protein.
- Plain corn tortillas.
- Bean burritos or enchiladas.
- Soft tacos made with grilled chicken or lean beef and rice.
- Mesquite-grilled chicken or seafood.
- Black bean soup.
- Gazpacho soup.
- Ceviche: seafood that has been marinated in lime juice and served in a spicy salsa mixture.
- Green corn tamales, enchiladas, and burritos (ask for them without cheese).
- Hot chili peppers, an excellent source of vitamins A and C, can be good for the body (if you can take the heat).

Also, take advantage of the abundant vegetables and fruits used in Mexican cooking: tomatoes, onions, squash, cabbage, corn, peas, potatoes, bananas, papaya, mango, guava, pineapple, oranges, and apples.

What to Avoid

Stay away from chimichangas and flautas, which are deep-fried tacos and burritos. Enchiladas made with cheese can be a fat disaster, as can chili rellenos when cheese is used. Tortilla chips, which usually contain at least 40 percent fat, and nachos, which have even more fat, are obvious extras to avoid. Guacamole is made from avocado, so the fat is monosaturated, but don't eat too much as it is calorie heavy. Avoid fried tortillas, refried beans cooked in lard, sour cream, jack cheese, and cilantro pesto (it contains nuts and oil).

INDIAN

Indian cookery is rich in vegetable protein. An abundant combination of vegetables, fruits, and herbs has made this traditional diet one of the healthiest. Many dishes include eggplant, okra, squash in dozens of varieties, green beans, tomatoes, cauliflower, peas, peppers, and a wide range of leafy greens, as well as legumes and potatoes. Over a hundred different fruits are part of this ancient diet, including apples, avocados, bananas, coconuts, dates, grapes, guavas, mangoes, oranges, and pomegranates. Seasonings such as mustard seed, turmeric, fenugreek, cinnamon, cloves, fresh ginger, garlic, and cilantro are also all used. Eighteen varieties of beans, peas, and lentils provide the protein in the diet. The many toppings, sauces, and marinades made of yogurt supply calcium.

There is no one Indian diet. Food choices vary from north to south and from the coast to the plains of the interior. Rice is a staple that is consumed throughout the country. Wheat is the other frequently consumed grain, though more in the north than in the south. The average Indian eats one-half pound of rice a day.

Chicken and lamb are the most common meats eaten. Pork is eaten in some western communities, and beef is eaten in the north. Fish and seafood tend to be eaten in the coastal regions of the east. Most people who live in the south are vegetarians. Although they use dairy products, eggs are avoided.

Boiling, stewing, and frying are the most common methods of cooking in the north while in the south steaming is preferred.

What to Eat

- Mulligatawny, a soup made with split peas, vegetables, herbs, and spices. Make sure the restaurant doesn't add cream.
- Dal rasam, a lentil soup. Make sure the restaurant doesn't add cream.

- Papadam is a bean wafer that is sometimes spiced with black pepper.
- Chapathi is a thin and dry bread made with whole wheat flour. Some restaurants put butter on chapathi, so ask for it without butter.
- Nan is another bread. It is unleavened and baked in a tandoor oven. Ask for it without butter.
- Any entree cooked in a tandoor oven is healthy, because the oven allows the fat to drip off. Chicken tandoor is a great choice, as are kabobs. They can be made from ground beef or lamb or cubes of meat. Make sure the meat is lean. Our experts told us that Indian restaurants routinely put butter on the kabobs right before serving. Just tell them you're allergic to butter!
- Fish tikka is fish marinated on a skewer and cooked in a tandoor. Shrimp is also cooked this way.
- Aloo palak is spinach with potatoes and spices.
- Paneer palak is homemade cottage cheese — usually a small amount — cooked with vegetables.
- Biriyani is a rice and vegetable dish made with raisins, saffron, and other spices. Try lamb, chicken, or shrimp.
- Rice pulao is a rice side dish with saffron and herbs.
- Vindaloo, a spicy dish influenced by the Portuguese, is made with shrimp, chicken, or beef. It should be cooked in a spicy sauce with little oil.
- Rogan josh, a sauce with onions, tomatoes, and spices, can be eaten with chicken, rice, or vegetables.

What to Avoid

Wahida Karmally, M.S., R.D., of Columbia Presbyterian Medical Center in New York says that you should be wary of anything fried, "particularly the appetizers." Deep-fried dishes to watch out for include pakori (vegetables), samosa (meat wrapped in dough), and bhatura (a bread). A high-fat paratha (a multilayered white-flour bread) is cooked with vegetable oil and topped with butter. If you try it, make it a little better by asking that no butter be added to the bread. Poori is a soft and fluffy white-flour bread that is deep-fried in vegetable oil. Look for the following words: *makkhani* means something in butter, and *malai* means cream. Curries are sometimes made with coconut, so ask for curry without coconut. Karmally warns, "A lot of restaurants put a chutney on the table with marinated onions or tomatoes as a side dish. The green or white salsa is called coconut chutney, and it is not good for you." Unfortunately, most restaurants in the United States use whole-fat yogurt in the refreshing drink lassi. Order it only if the chef can make it for you with low-fat yogurt.

CHINESE

Most Chinese people remain in the province where they were born and maintain their traditional eating patterns. They eat a diet of fruits, grains, and vegetables, with very little meat or dairy products. This diet is high in fiber and low in cholesterol and fat. Cooking is done with a vegetable oil, such as peanut, which is low in saturated fat. In 1991, Dr. T. Colin Campbell of Cornell University determined that the traditional Chinese diet is among the world's best for preventing heart disease and some cancers. The rate of colon cancer among the Chinese is half that among Americans; the rate of heart disease among Chinese men is one-seventeenth that among American men; and the rate of breast cancer in China is one-fifth the rate here.

Cantonese, Mandarin, Hunan, and Szechuan are the predominant styles of Chinese cooking in the United States. They differ in the degree of spiciness and use of staples. All the diets have in common rice, pastas, and noodles. Rice flour, bean starch, and milled wheat are all used in the production of noodle products. The greatest variety in the Chinese diet is found in the 2,000 different vegetables consumed. In Canton, the southeastern coastal area, the number of dishes ranges up to 50,000. Other basic foods are freshwater fish and seafood, chicken, pork, and duck. Beef is a relatively new part of the Chinese diet. It is expensive and still used sparingly in everyday eating.

The Chinese cook small amounts of meat with lots of vegetables, rice, and noodles. This is the opposite of the standard American meal — a large piece of meat and a tiny side order of vegetables.

Stir-frying is the method of choice in China. Food is fast-cooked in a wok, which helps retain the vitamins and minerals of fresh vegetables. Steaming is another healthy method that the Chinese use to enhance the natural flavor of their dishes.

This section on Chinese food is longer than the others for two reasons. First, the Chinese have the best-documented therapeutic effect from foods of any culture studied. Second, Chinese take-out and restaurants are the most popular in America. Most Americans order Chinese food because they believe it is healthy. Although Chinese food in China is healthy, Chinese food in America makes a hamburger outlet look like nutrition's holy grail.

What to Eat

Choose dishes that are boiled, steamed, or lightly stir-fried in vegetable oil rather than sauteed. Try vegetable dishes, noodles, and steamed brown rice. Rice is the core of the diet in the south. Noodles, bread, and dumplings made from wheat are the rule in the temperate north. Bok choy and other forms of Chinese cabbage — perhaps the most widely consumed vegetables in the world — are cruciferous, high in vitamin C, and contribute to general good health. Vegetables such as cabbage, bean sprouts, water chestnuts, snow peas, broccoli, and bamboo shoots are healthy additions that provide flavor, as do exotic mushrooms and tofu. Good soup choices are the thin Chinese soups like sweet and sour and wonton.

Healthy dishes to ask for include:

- Steamed dumplings (filled with vegetables, not meat).
- Steamed or braised fish or scallops with black bean sauce.
- Chicken or eggplant steamed or braised.
- Stir-fried vegetables with chicken, shrimp, or tofu.
- Steamed crabmeat with ginger.
- Shrimp with vegetables, black bean sauce, or garlic sauce.

For dessert, have fresh fruit: sliced oranges, melon, pineapple, lychees (fresh or dried). You can have the fortune inside the fortune cookies, says Gordon Wardlaw, but skip the cookies.

What to Avoid

Avoid MSG (monosodium glutamate). It's loaded with salt and chemicals and is suspected of attacking the nervous system. If a menu doesn't state that the restaurant doesn't use MSG, you're almost certainly going to get it in your food. U.S. versions of Chinese fare regrettably emphasize meats and sauces. American Chinese restaurants can serve food terribly high in fat. Specific dishes to avoid include:

- Fried egg rolls and dumplings.
- Sesame noodles.
- Fried rice, which is also heavy and difficult to digest.
- Peking duck.
- Anything "crispy" or "batter-coated" (both terms indicate deep frying).
- Dishes heavy on nuts, such as kung pao chicken.
- Heavy meat dishes, such as pork, beef, and some duck dishes, are overloaded with animal fats.
- Limit egg foo yung dishes as well as all foods made with lobster sauces. They contain egg yolks and are high in cholesterol.
- Avoid fatty items such as duck and fatty pork (ribs).
- American Chinese dishes tend to contain too much soy sauce, which is loaded with sodium. Ask your waiter to make sure the chef doesn't drench your meal in soy sauce. One expert recommends rice vinegar as a good substitute.

The Center for Science in the Public Interest conducted an investigation of Chinese food sold in the United States Its conclusion? Chinese food is not a healthy cuisine as prepared in many U.S. restaurants. A typical carton of kung pao chicken has as much fat as four McDonald's quarter-pounders! Here are the fifteen most popular

Chinese Dishes	Amount of Dish	Amount of Rice	Calories	Fat (g)	Cholesterol (mg)	Sodium (mg)
Szechuan shrimp	2⅔ cups	1⅓ cups	927	19	336	2,457
Stir-fried vegetables	2⅔ cups	1⅓ cups	746	19	0	2,153
Shrimp with garlic sauce	1⅓ cups	1⅓ cups	945	27	307	2,951
Hunan tofu	2⅔ cups	1⅓ cups	907	28	0	2,316
Chicken chow mein	3⅔ cups	1⅓ cups	1,005	32	205	2,446
House fried rice	4 cups	——	1,484	50	346	2,682
House lo mein	5 cups	——	1,059	36	175	3,460
Hot and sour soup	1 cup	——	112	4	129	1,088
Orange (crispy) beef	2⅔ cups	1⅓ cups	1,766	66	296	3,135
General Tso's chicken	3⅔ cups	1⅓ cups	1,597	59	342	3,148
Beef with broccoli	2⅔ cups	1⅓ cups	1,175	46	228	3,146
Sweet and sour pork	2⅔ cups	1⅓ cups	1,613	71	118	818
Kung pao chicken	3⅔ cups	1⅓ cups	1,620	76	277	2,608
Mu shu pork	2⅔ cups	1⅓ cups	1,228	64	465	2,593
Egg roll	1 roll	——	190	11	7	463
Extras						
Soy sauce	1 tbsp	——	11	0	0	1,029
Fortune cookie	1	——	30	0	0	22
Soup noodles	½ cup	——	150	8	0	300
Chow mein noodles	½ cup	——	119	7	0	99

Chinese dishes. You can see many are loaded with enormous amounts of fat, cholesterol, calories, and sodium.

How to Make It Better

Here's what CSPI suggests to make dining Chinese a healthier experience.

Add Rice. The more rice you put on your plate, the more portions you create and therefore the less sodium and fat each portion contains. That kung pao chicken without the rice averaged 1,275 calories, 75 g of fat (13 of them saturated), and more than 2,600 mg of sodium. But if you add one cup of rice to every cup of kung pao and then divide it into two-cup portions, each will have about 653 calories, 23 g of fat (4 of them saturated), and 791 mg of sodium.

Chinese Dishes	Amount of Dish	Amount of Rice	Calories	Fat (g)	Cholesterol (mg)	Sodium (mg)
Stir-fried vegetables	1 cup	1 cup	400	6	0	717
Szechuan shrimp	1 cup	1 cup	509	8	140	1,025
House lo mein	1 cup	1 cup	497	8	38	752
House fried rice	1 cup	1 cup	605	12	79	610
Chicken chow mein	1 cup	1 cup	450	9	57	681
Hunan tofu	1 cup	1 cup	454	9	0	772
Shrimp with garlic sauce	1 cup	1 cup	552	13	146	1,405
General Tso's chicken	1 cup	1 cup	657	19	107	983
Beef with broccoli	1 cup	1 cup	563	16	81	1,124
Orange (crispy) beef	1 cup	1 cup	724	21	95	1,010
Kung pao chicken	1 cup	1 cup	653	23	84	791
Sweet and sour pork	1 cup	1 cup	817	31	51	355
Mu shu pork	1 cup	1 cup	574	22	162	903

Reprinted/adapted from Nutrition Action Healthletter (1875 Connecticut Avenue, N.W., Washington, D.C. 20009-5728).

Ask for Steamed Veggies. American Chinese food emphasizes meat or chicken. The key is to put the emphasis on the vegetables. Ask for a side order of steamed vegetables and add them to your dish.

Do the "Forklift." CSPI claims that this is how the Chinese eat. Use your fork (or chopsticks) to lift the food out of the sauce and onto your bowl of rice.

- Place egg rolls in a napkin to sop up grease.
- Instead of mu shu pork, order mu shu vegetables with no egg.
- Kung pao chicken is usually loaded with peanuts, sometimes nearly a cup per dish. Ask for no more than three tablespoons of nuts.
- Most of the fat in sweet-and-sour pork is in the breading. You can remove the fat by taking off the breading.
- With any beef and vegetable dish, ask for less beef and more vegetable.

- If the restaurant batter-fries the chicken or beef in a dish, peel the coating off.
- Instead of lo mein with chicken, shrimp, beef, or pork, order vegetable lo mein and mix it with rice.
- Never order an entree and then put it on top of fried rice. If it's your main dish, ask for vegetable fried rice with no egg, and mix it with steamed rice.
- If your dish comes with fried noodles, ask that they be left out.
- Instead of stir-fried vegetables, try them steamed and sprinkled lightly with soy sauce. Be careful of the soy sauce — every teaspoon costs you 350 mg of sodium.

Chapter 9

Grazing

EATING ON THE RUN IS WHAT HUMANS HAVE DONE FOR MILLIONS OF years. Many nomadic people continue to eat that way today, including men who live on airplanes. True nomads have spectacularly low cholesterol levels and little heart disease. They undertake prolonged, low-intensity exercise and eat almost continuously. Both measures keep their metabolism high, so their bodies remain lean, calorie-burning machines. But indiscriminate grazing on burgers, pizza, doughnuts, soft drinks, hot salted pretzels, and hot dogs during a wild and frantic day in the industrial world can be a nutritional disaster.

Conventional Wisdom:
> *Eating between meals is bad for you.*

New Paradigm:
> *Grazing is the best, most natural way to eat . . . if you know what to look for.*

A poor grazer ingests whatever comes across his path. A good grazer knows what quantity and quality of food to aim for. The 1992 U.S. Department of Agriculture's recommended food groups provide a good guide for grazing. Just aim for the recommended number of servings during a day and you're assured of getting the minimum amount of nutrients you need. Foods in these groups are far from being nutritionally equal. Grazing from the food lists provided throughout this chapter will deliver superior nutrition that even the most expensive supplements will be challenged to meet. Here is what counts as one serving and the number of servings to aim for in three different calorie ranges.

What Counts As a Serving
BREADS, CEREALS, RICE, AND PASTA
    1 slice of bread
    ½ cup of cooked rice or pasta
    ½ cup of cooked cereal
    1 ounce of ready-to-eat cereal
VEGETABLES
    ½ cup of chopped raw or cooked vegetables
    1 cup of leafy raw vegetables
FRUITS
    1 piece of fruit or melon wedge
    ¾ cup of juice
    ½ cup of canned fruit
    ¼ cup of dried fruit
MILK, YOGURT, AND CHEESE
    1 cup of milk or yogurt
    1½ to 2 ounces of cheese
MEAT, POULTRY, FISH, DRY BEANS, EGGS, AND NUTS
    2½ to 3 ounces of cooked lean meat, poultry, fish
    Count ½ cup of cooked beans, or 1 egg, or 2 tablespoons of peanut butter as 1 ounce of lean meat (about ⅓ serving)

1,600 Calories
Bread, cereal, rice, pasta, and baked goods: *6 servings*
Vegetables and beans: *3 servings*
Fruits: *2 servings*
Dairy foods: *2 to 3 servings*
Fish, poultry, meat, nuts, and eggs: *5 servings*

2,200 Calories

Bread, cereal, rice, pasta, and baked goods: *9 servings*

Vegetables and beans: *4 servings*

Fruits: *3 servings*

Dairy foods: *2 to 3 servings*

Fish, poultry, meats, nuts, and eggs: *6 servings*

2,800 Calories

Bread, cereal, rice, pasta and baked goods: *11 servings*

Vegetables and beans: *5 servings*

Fruits: *4 servings*

Dairy foods: *2 to 3 servings*

Fish, poultry, meat, nuts, and eggs: *7 servings*

If you think real men don't weigh food, talk to professional weight-training coach John Parrillo. The way that bodybuilders get to look exactly as they want is through knowing exactly how many calories they eat. Now, I don't mean you need to become obsessed with weighing every scrap of food that goes into your mouth. However, each time you eat a food for the first time after reading this chapter, measure it. Get a sense of portion size. Within a few weeks you'll know precisely what you're eating without the scales or measuring cups.

THE BEST FOODS

Remember that different foods from the same food group are far from equal. Let's say you select iceberg lettuce from the vegetable group. This lettuce has almost no nutrition, whereas a sweet potato is stuffed full of nutrients. For this reason I have included lists that rank the best choices for vegetables, fruits, grains, beans, and dairy products. Chapter 6, "Get Hard," ranks proteins by quality and fat content. Identify five to ten foods you really like from the top of each of these lists and memorize them. Try to choose them whenever you graze.

I'm grateful to the Center for Science in the Public Interest, which generously made most of the following lists available.

VEGETABLES

CSPI scored each vegetable by adding up its percent of the USRDA for six nutrients plus fiber. Here's an example: one medium raw carrot has 405 percent of the USRDA for vitamin A (405 points), 11 percent for vitamin C (11 points), 9 percent for fiber (9 points), 3 percent for folic acid (3 points), and 2 percent each for calcium, iron, and copper (6 points). That adds up to a total of 434 points. If no number was available (NA) for a nutrient (folic acid or copper for leaf lettuce, for example), it was assigned a value of 0. That could make the scores of some vegetables lower than they should be. CSPI says, "That was okay with us because vitamin A (which occurs in vegetables as beta-carotene), vitamin C, and folic acid are the nutrients most people need to get from vegetables (or fruit)."

While there are no vegetables that are bad for you, some are pretty weak players. In an article in a 1991 edition of *Nutrition Action Healthletter,* CSPI's newsletter, Bonnie Liebman writes, "Many of America's favorite vegetables — like iceberg lettuce and celery — are among the least nutritious. . . . The typical 'salad,' for example, combines some of the least nutritious vegetables. Its base is iceberg lettuce, now the second most popular American vegetable after potatoes. Eat a whole cup of iceberg and you get ten percent of the U.S. Recommended Daily Allowance (USRDA) for . . . well, nothing! Likewise for salad vegetables like cucumbers, alfalfa sprouts, and raw mushrooms. Only tomatoes exceed ten percent of the USRDA for vitamin C — if you eat half a tomato."

According to the article, celery, beets, and onions may be fun to eat, but nutrients are not their forte. Green beans barely get by with some vitamin C. For a salad, spinach or romaine lettuce is a much better pick. So next time the waiter asks what kind of salad you'd like, take a pass unless the salad is made with a dark leafy green, since a fatty dressing on iceberg lettuce with celery is worse than nothing at all. Instead, choose one or two big-winner vegetables with the main course.

Which ones are the big winners? The sweet potato is the king of the vegetable kingdom. A sweet potato supplies half the USRDA for vitamin C and an impressive 3.4 grams of fiber, even without the skin. Carrots are second, with more than four times the USRDA for beta-carotene. "Spinach, collards, kale, dandelion greens, mustard greens, and Swiss chard are the decathletes of the vegetable kingdom," says Bonnie. I've found lots of good news in this list, since I'd far rather have sweet potatoes, carrots, collard greens, and broccoli than cabbage, cauliflower, and mushrooms. I've memorized my favorite ten out of the top of the list and use them for grazing from our CBS cafeteria, salad bars, grocery stores, and hors d'oeuvres trays.

Vegetable (½ cup cooked unless noted)	Score[1]	Vitamin A	Vitamin C	Folic Acid	Iron	Copper	Calcium
Sweet potato, no skin (1)	582	†	†	★		†	
Carrot, raw (1)	434	†	†				
Carrots	408	†				★	
Spinach	241	†	†	†	†	★	†
Collard greens, frozen	181	†	†	†	★		†
Red pepper, raw (½)	166	†	†				
Kale	161	†	†			★	★
Dandelion greens	156	†	†	NA	★	NA	★
Spinach, raw (1 cup)	152	†	†	†	★		★
Broccoli	145	†	†	†			
Brussels sprouts	128	†	†	†	★		
Broccoli, frozen	127	†	†	†			★
Potato, baked, with skin (1)	114	NA	†	★	†	†	
Mixed vegetables, frozen	111	†	★				
Winter squash	110	†	†	★		★	
Swiss chard	105	†	†	NA	†	NA	★
Broccoli, raw	100	†	†	★			
Snow peas	90		†	NA	★		
Mustard greens	85	†	†	NA		NA	★
Kohlrabi	82		†	NA		NA	
Romaine lettuce (1 cup)	78	†	†	†		NA	
Cauliflower	77		†	★			

Vegetable (½ cup cooked unless noted)	Score[1]	Vitamin A	Vitamin C	Folic Acid	Iron	Copper	Calcium
Asparagus	75	†	†	†		★	
Green peppers, raw (½)	67	★	†				
Potato, baked, no skin (1)	67	NA	†			†	
Parsley, raw (¼ cup)	66	†	†	★	★		
Green peas, frozen	64	†	†	†	★	★	
Avocado, California (½)	63	†	†	†	★	†	
Okra	61	★	†	†			★
Collard greens	57	†	†				
Endive, raw (1 cup)	56	†	★	†			
Parsnips	53		†	†		†	
Rutabaga	48		†				
Cabbage	47		†				
Artichoke (½)	46		†	★		★	
Mushrooms	43		★		★	†	
Cabbage, raw	39		†	★			
Corn	39		★	†			
Boston lettuce, raw (1 cup)	38	†	★	†			NA
Green beans	37	★	†	★			
Tomato, raw (½)	37	★	†				
Beets	32		★	†			
Summer squash	31	★	★	★		★	
Corn, frozen	23			★			
Lettuce, iceberg (1 cup)	22			★			
Radishes, raw (¼ cup)	17		†				
Celery, raw (1 stalk)	14		★				
Onions, raw (¼ cup)	14						
Eggplant	12						
Alfalfa sprouts (½ cup)	11						
Cucumber, raw	11						
Mushrooms, raw	10						
Garlic, raw (1 clove)	3					NA	

[1] There is no USRDA for fiber, so CSPI made up its own, 25 grams, and factored it into the scores in the table.

★Contains between 5 and 9 percent of the USRDA.

†Contains at least 10 percent of the USRDA.

Blanks indicate less than 5 percent USRDA.

NA means data not available.

Reprinted/adapted from Nutrition Action Healthletter (1875 Connecticut Avenue, N.W., Washington, D.C. 20009-5728).

FRUITS

Papaya and cantaloupe top the list of best fruits. Each provides almost a complete daily dose of vitamin A and C with a hefty helping of potassium. Grapes have a respectable, but unimpressive, 10 percent of the USRDA for vitamin C. Dry them into raisins and you'll have lots less. Canning destroys vitamin C but not vitamin A, which is more stable. Does an apple a day keep the doctor away? You stand a much better shot at staying beyond his clutches with over a dozen other fruits, from strawberries to kiwis and apricots.

Fruit	Score	Calories	Vitamin A	Vitamin C	Folic Acid	Potassium[1]	Fiber[1]
Papaya (½)	252	59	†	†	NA	†	†
Cantaloupe (¼)	213	47	†	†	★	†	
Strawberries (1 cup)	186	45		†	★	★	†
Oranges (1)	169	62	★	†	★	★	†
Tangerines (2)	168	74	†	†	★	★	†
Kiwis (1)	154	46		†	NA	★	†
Mango (½)	153	68	†	†	NA		★
Apricots (4)	143	68	†	†		†	†
Persimmons (1)	134	118	†	†		★	†
Watermelon (2 cups)	122	100	†	†		†	★
Raspberries (1 cup)	117	61		†	NA	★	†
Grapefruit, red or pink (½)	103	37	★	†			
Blackberries (1 cup)	101	74		†	NA	★	†
Apricots, dried (10)	97	83	†			†	†
Grapefruit, white (½)	84	39		†		★	
Honeydew melon (¹⁄₁₀)	81	46		†	NA	†	
Peaches (2)	77	74	†	†		★	†
Pineapple (1 cup)	77	77		†		★	★

Fruit	Score	Calories	Vitamin A	Vitamin C	Folic Acid	Potassium[1]	Fiber[1]
Star fruit (1)	73	42	†	†	NA	★	NA
Blueberries (1 cup)	68	82		†			†
Cherries, sweet (1 cup)	64	104	★	†		★	★
Nectarines (1)	64	67	†	†		★	★
Pomegranates (1)	61	104	NA	†	NA	†	†
Bananas (1)	60	105		†	★	†	★
Plums (2)	60	72	★	†		★	★
Prunes, dried (5)	59	101	†			★	†
Apples, with skin (1)	58	124		†		★	†
Boysenberries (1 cup)	57	66		★	†	★	NA
Pears (1)	48	98		†		★	†
Grapes, green (60)	46	90		†		★	
Peaches, canned in juice	43	68	†	★	NA	★	
Apples, no skin (1)	42	111		†		★	†
Pineapple, canned in juice	40	70		†	NA		
Figs, dried (2)	39	95				★	†
Currants, dried (¼ cup)	36	102				★	
Rhubarb, cooked (½ cup)	36	139		★			NA
Raisins (¼ cup, packed)	35	124				★	★

Fruit	Score	Calories	Vitamin A	Vitamin C	Folic Acid	Potassium[1]	Fiber[1]
Dates (5)	30	114				★	★
Pears, canned in juice	16	76			NA		NA

[1]*CSPI made up its own RDA for fiber (25 g) and potassium (3,500 mg).*
★*Contains between 5 and 9 percent of the USRDA.*
†*Contains at least 10 percent of the USRDA.*
Blanks indicate less than 5 percent USRDA.
NA means data not available.
Reprinted/adapted from Nutrition Action Healthletter *(1875 Connecticut Avenue, N.W., Washington, D.C. 20009-5728).*

BEANS

Beans are at the heart of several of the world's healthiest diets. They're a rich source of carbohydrates, protein, fiber, minerals, and vitamins. The chart shows how they score.

Bean (1 cup cooked)	Score	Fiber	Folic Acid	Magnesium	Iron	Copper	Zinc
Soybeans	300	○	★	○	●	○	★
Pinto beans	287	●	●	○	○	★	★
Chickpeas (garbanzos, ceci)	286	●	●	★	○	○	★
Lentils	285	●	●	★	○	★	★
Cranberry beans	278	●	●	★	★	★	★
Black-eyed peas (cowpeas)	273	○	●	★	○	★	★
Pink beans	269	○	●	○	★	★	★
Navy beans	266	●	●	○	○	○	★
Black beans (turtle beans)	265	●	●	○	★	★	★
Small white beans	263	●	●	○	○	★	★
White beans	253	○	○	○	○	○	★
Lima beans, baby	252	●	●	★	★	★	★
Kidney beans, all types	243	○	●	★	○	★	★
Adzuki beans	238	○	●	★	★	○	★
Great Northern beans	228	●	○	★	★	★	★
Mung beans	226	●	●	★	★	★	★
Lima beans, large	224	●	○	★	★	★	★
Broad beans (fava beans)	197	○	○	★	★	★	★

Bean (1 cup cooked)	Score	Fiber	Folic Acid	Magnesium	Iron	Copper	Zinc
Peas, split (green)	192	●	○	★	★	★	★
Tofu, raw, firm (4 oz)	178	†	†	○	●	★	★
Tofu, raw, regular	109	†	†	○	○	★	†

●Contains at least 50 percent of the USRDA.
○Contains between 25 and 49 percent of the USRDA.
★Contains between 10 and 24 percent of the USRDA.
†Contains less than 10 percent of the USRDA.
Reprinted/adapted from Nutrition Action Healthletter (1875 Connecticut Avenue, N.W., Washington, D.C. 20009-5728).

GRAINS

Many men underrate grains because too many of us eat them in the form of white flour found in pizza, bagels, pastas, and bread products. Those highly processed foods have little natural nutrient value. However, minimally processed grains are a food bonanza. Many nutritionists consider whole grains the most valuable of all foods, rich in protein, carbohydrates, fiber, vitamins, and minerals. What's more, this is the bulk of all the food you eat in a day, double to triple the number of servings of any other food group. Unfortunately, processing strips away the layers that contain protein, fiber, and B vitamins. A lot of men believe that grains are fattening, but eaten as whole grains they are highly satisfactory hunger quenchers with terrific nutrient value. If every time you're tempted to eat a fatty, sugary junk-food treat you reach for a whole-grain product instead, you'll drop weight like a stone.

This past year I've become a big fan of grains I had never heard of before, like amaranth, food of the Aztecs, and quinoa, used in Bolivia over 3,000 years ago. Around our house, we've found that substituting whole wheat spaghetti for white–flour spaghetti detracts in no way from the taste and satisfaction of the meal, supplies super-nutrients, and doesn't leave you hungry hours later. Here's how they rank.

Grain (5 oz cooked)	Score	Fiber	Magnesium	B₆	Zinc	Copper	Iron
Quinoa xxx	73	★	●	—	★	●	●
Macaroni or spaghetti, whole wheat	69	●	●	★	★	●	★
Amaranth xxx	66	●	●	—	★	●	●
Buckwheat groats xxx	64	●	●	★	★	●	★
Spaghetti, spinach	61	NA	●	★	●	●	★
Bulgar xxx	60	●	●	★	★	★	★
Barley, pearled xxx	59	●	★	★	★	★	●
Wild rice xxx	58	●	●	●	●	★	★
Millet xxx	53	★	●	★	★	●	★
Brown rice xxx	51	●	●	●	★	★	—
Triticale xxx	47	●	●	—	★	★	—
Spaghetti	42	●	★	—	★	★	●
Wheat berries xxx	41	●	★	—	★	★	★
Macaroni	39	★	★	—	★	★	●
Kamut	37	NA	●	—	★	★	★
Oats, rolled	33	●	★	—	★	—	★
Spelt	33	●	●	NA	NA	—	★
White rice, converted	26	—	—	—	—	★	★
Couscous	23	★	—	—	—	—	—
White rice, instant	18	—	—	—	—	★	★
Soba noodles	12	NA	—	—	—	—	—
Corn grits	10	—	—	—	—	—	★

xxx or "Best Bite" designates the best overall choices.
●Contains at least 10 percent of the USRDA.
★Contains between 5 and 9 percent of the USRDA.
—Contains less than 5 percent USRDA.
NA indicates data not available.
Reprinted/adapted from Nutrition Action Healthletter (1875 Connecticut Avenue, N.W., Washington, D.C. 20009-5728).

DAIRY PRODUCTS

Dairy products contain the highest grade of protein available. Food processing allows producers to offer a wide range of products stripped of the fats. The following list of products is ranked for high protein quality and calcium content and low fat. It was formulated by sports nutritionist Liz Applegate, Ph.D., nutrition columnist, *Runner's World* magazine.

Dairy product	Amount	Calories	% Fat Calories	Saturated Fat (g)	Protein (g)	Calcium (mg)
Plain nonfat yogurt	1 cup	140	0	0	14	499
Skim milk	1 cup	86	0	0	8	302
Low-fat plain yogurt	1 cup	159	23	3	13	458
1% milk	1 cup	102	26	2	8	300
Nonfat vanilla yogurt	1 cup	195	5	<1	12	432
Buttermilk	1 cup	99	18	1	8	285
Low-fat vanilla yogurt	1 cup	209	13	2	12	418
Nonfat fruit-flavored yogurt	1 cup	200	0	0	9	333
Chocolate (1% fat) milk	1 cup	158	11	1	8	287
Low-fat fruit-flavored yogurt	1 cup	249	11	2	10	347
Nonfat cottage cheese	1 cup	203	19	1	28	138
Mozzarella cheese	1 oz	71	5	3	7	181
Monterey Jack cheese	1 oz	80	67	3	8	250
Nonfat frozen yogurt	½ cup	100	0	0	4	130
Reduced-fat cheese	1 oz	73	53	2	6	214
Low-fat frozen yogurt	½ cup	110	16	1	4	120
Parmesan cheese	1 oz	111	59	5	10	336
Part-skim ricotta cheese	½ cup	171	51	6	14	337
Provolone cheese	1 oz	100	66	5	7	214
Gouda cheese	1 oz	101	68	5	7	198

SUPERSUPPLEMENTS

Many men completely miss out on the five-a-day fruits and vege-tables because they are hard to prepare and time-consuming to eat. They rely instead on supplements, because they're easy and fast.

I interviewed scientists at the Center for Science in the Public Interest about this problem, and they suggested a solution called the Vita-Mixer. I had visions of the juicers that have been so popular over the last several years on late-night TV. CSPI reiterated that these are essentially worthless because they leave behind the pulp, which contains most of the nutrients. If you squeeze your own orange juice, you leave two-thirds of the vitamin C behind in the pulp! Save the pulp and you get vitamins and much less rise in blood sugar. I remained skeptical until I saw the Vita-Mixer's secret — a 37,000-rpm, nearly two-horsepower lawn mower–quality engine that can blast pulp, fiber, and even seeds into smithereens. Standard juicers leave juice so gritty you may find it unpleasant to drink. The Vita-Mixer produces a smooth puree.

The manufacturer claims that all the nutrients are retained and that the machine liberates more of them than even our own digestive systems can. The machine blasted wheat germ into a pharmaceutical-grade powder. It took oranges and grapefruits with their skins and ground them to the point that there were no seeds or rinds left. The smoothie had no grit, no pulp, no aftertaste. When it came to concocting a megadose of antioxidants, it was like painting a house with a spray gun instead of a one-inch paintbrush. I ordered two — one for home and one for the office — determined to invent a way to make an antioxidant cocktail that was quick, easy, and tasty.

Dr. Charles H. Hennekens, the John Snow Professor of medicine, ambulatory care, and prevention at Harvard Medical School, chief of preventive medicine at Brigham and Women's Hospital in Boston, and chair of the Worldwide Antioxidants Trialists Collaboration, indicated that supplements alone may not cut it in terms of getting the right disease-preventing compounds. Why? Because the extraction process leaves behind hundreds of different components of real food, the most critical of which are called phytochemicals, key disease-prevention chemicals. The absence of phytochemicals may be why antioxidant supplements alone aren't nearly as effective as whole foods. Here's an example. An apple has 389 phytochemicals. Leave out the skin and you miss many of those phytochemicals. So far, 59 phytochemicals have been identified as known cell protectors and detoxifiers, but there are 102,000 more. Many experts recommend taking advantage of those phytochemicals now. Phytochemicals are called the quintessence of nutrition and may be the hot new nutrients of the 1990s. A study reported in the medical journal *The Lancet* in 1993 showed that one class of phytochemicals, called bioflavenoids, protected Dutch men from heart disease. With the Vita-Mixer you can produce your own phytochemical-rich cocktails. Here are several sample recipes.

◆

Duke's Mix

Dr. James Duke, an economic botanist at the USDA, pioneered the idea of food as medicine. This is the recipe for his favorite antioxidant cocktail.

2 to 4 fresh or canned tomatoes

1 to 2 sweet red or green peppers

hot pepper to taste — any type of jalapeño is fine — for the antioxidant capsaicin

1 whole onion with skin (it's the richest source of the antioxidant quercetin)

½ cup kale and/or turnip greens or collards

1 to 4 fresh carrots

1 cup purslane, a common weed available at most farmers markets

1 to 2 spears broccoli

Mix to your liking.

◆

Super Fruit Juice
(provided by the Vita-Mix Corporation)

¼ ripe banana

¼ cup cantaloupe

¼ cup strawberries

¼ orange, including white part of peel

¼ cup red seedless grapes

¼ cup Mori-Nu Lite Tofu

¼ cup carrots, cut in 1-inch lengths

1¼ apples, seeded

2 dates, pitted

2 prunes, pitted

1 cup ice

Speed: high
Time: 1½ minutes
Yield: 2 cups

◆

Hot Vegetable Super Juice
(provided by the Vita-Mix Corporation)
¼ cup baked potato, with skin
¼ cup cooked sweet potato, peeled
¼ cup carrots, cut in 1-inch lengths
¼ cup celery, cut in 1-inch lengths
¼ cup broccoli, raw or cooked
1 Italian plum tomato
1 clove garlic
1 small green onion, including roots and top
1 spinach leaf
1 teaspoon flax seed
1¼ cups hot water

Speed: high
Time: 2 minutes
Yield: 3 cups

Seasoning suggestions include pepper, hot pepper, lime, broth or bouillon, Mrs. Dash, rosemary, or other herbs.

SUPERSNACKS

Building an Arsenal of Superfoods

Most active men just don't have the time to drag long food lists into stores, check the label of every food, or become big-league chefs. We're also creatures of habit, eating a pretty limited number of foods and meals. So just as it's important to learn to eat ten new super-healthful meals, it's important to construct your list of minimeals and processed health foods to eat on the run. Here's what to look for.

1. Slow-burning carbohydrates.
2. High-quality protein.

3. Fiber.
4. Minerals and vitamins.

The following list offers foods that have no preservatives, artificial colors, artificial flavors, refined or synthetic sugars or sweeteners (including brown sugar, fructose, dextrose, aspartame, saccharin, or sorbitol), no cottonseed, coconut, or palm-kernel oils, and no hydrogenated oils. In most of the products containing flour, the flour is mostly composed of whole-grain flour.

Several times a month take a trip to a high-quality health food store or whole-food supermarket. Stockpile your purchases where they're needed most: in your office, luggage, briefcase, knapsack, desk, and car. When you are tempted to eat from a vending machine or airline food tray, reach for any of the following or choose your own superfoods based on these samples.

Alvardo St. Bakery Sprouted Wheat Bagels
Serving: 1 bagel
Fat: 1 gram
Calories: 250

Pro:
• Great slow-burning carbohydrate
• Good protein but not a complete protein — lacks lycine
• Low fat
• Contains organically grown wheat berries

Lifestream Essene Sprouted Grain Loaf
Serving: 2 ounces
Fat: none
Calories: 140

Pro:
• Great source of protein from soybeans, whole wheat, and oats
• Great source of soluble and insoluble fiber from the oats, whole wheat, barley, buckwheat, and millet

- Nutrient-dense; high in thiamin and iron
- Very slow burning carbohydrate from the many grains
- Organic

Food for Life Fat-free Blueberry Muffins
Serving: 1 muffin
Fat: none
Calories: 40

Pro:
- Very low in calories
- Good slow-burning carbohydrate from the whole wheat flour
- Good protein from the wheat and some from egg whites
- Good source of insoluble fiber from the unprocessed wheat bran

Ancient Quinoa Harvest Pasta
Serving: 2 ounces dry pasta
Fat: 2 grams
Calories: 180

Pro:
- Good source of fiber from the quinoa and corn flour
- Fat comes from the corn, but it's natural, not added, and is unsaturated
- A slow-burning carbohydrate
- Good source of riboflavin and thiamin
- Good source of protein from the quinoa and corn flour, which is a better-quality protein than from a lot of grains but still not a complete protein
- No added sugar

Arrowhead Mills 100% Valencia Peanut Butter
Serving: 2 tablespoons
Fat: 15 grams
Calories: 200

Pro:
- Good source of protein, but not a complete protein
- A slow-burning carbohydrate
- No sodium
- No hydrogenated oils
- Great when combined sparingly with whole-grain breads

Con:
- High in fat and calories

American Prairie Organic Porridge Oats
Serving: ½ cup rolled oats
Fat: 2.5 grams
Calories: 160

Pro:
- Complex carbohydrate from the oats
- Low in fat
- No sodium
- Good source of iron
- Good source of protein, but not a complete protein
- Good source of soluble fiber
- No simple sugar

Guiltless Gourmet No Oil Tortilla Chips
Serving: 22 chips
Fat: 1.5 grams
Calories: 110

Pro:
- Short ingredient list: yellow corn, water, and lime
- Baked not fried
- Very low in fat; much less than other tortilla chips
- Good fiber for a snack
- A slow-burning carbohydrate
- A complete protein if eaten with a (preferably no-fat) bean dip

Health Valley Fat-free Fruit Bars

Serving: 1 bar

Fat: none

Calories: 140

Pro:

- Slow-burning carbohydrate from the organic oats and brown rice
- Fairly good source of fiber from the organic oats, brown rice, and blend of oat bran, wheat bran, amaranth, rye, barley, and corn
- Good source of iron

Con:

- Simple sugars from various juice concentrates
- Not a complete protein

Ak-Mak Crackers

Serving: 5 crackers

Fat: 2.27 grams

Calories: 116

Pro:

- 100 percent stone-ground wheat
- A slow-burning carbohydrate made with whole wheat flour
- Low fat; added sesame oil, which is unsaturated
- Good source of fiber
- Good amount of protein, although it's incomplete

Con:

- Fairly high sodium
- Not a good source of vitamins and minerals

Taste Adventures Navy Bean Soup

Serving: 6 ounces (four servings per container)

Fat: 5 grams

Calories: 111

Pro:

- Slow-burning carbohydrate
- Good source of protein from the navy beans

- Good source of soluble fiber
- Good source of iron

Amy's Organic Beans and Rice Burrito
Serving: 1 burrito or 170 grams
Fat: 5 grams
Calories: 250

Pro:
- Complete protein from the pinto beans, whole wheat flour, and brown rice
- Very little fat
- Good source of fiber
- Made with a little safflower oil, which is unsaturated

Baldwin Hill Sesame Bread
Serving: 2 ounces
Fat: 2 grams
Calories: 138

Pro:
- Slow-burning carbohydrate
- Good protein from the whole wheat, although not a complete protein
- Very little fat, mostly from the sesame seed
- Good source of fiber

Fantastic Foods Rice and Beans
Serving: 1 container
Fat: 2 grams
Calories: 210

Pro:
- Slow-burning carbohydrate from the brown rice
- Good source of protein from the beans

- Good source of soluble fiber
- Good source of iron

Con:
- High sodium

Look for other Fantastic Foods as a great source of slow-burning complex carbos and vegetarian protein.

Chapter 10

Be a Watchdog

IN NEARLY EVERY AIRPLANE, CAFETERIA, DINING ROOM, AND RESTAURANT in America, the "food police" routinely scold us for making poor nutritional choices whenever we move food in the general direction of our mouths. But like the self-deputized sheriff who couldn't shoot straight, the food police aren't just overbearing, they're often just plain wrong, espousing the latest popular misconceptions about new killer foods. Make no mistake, there is good reason for the emergence of the food police. Food shopping in America is a damned tricky business fraught with error and outright fraud, but your best protection is becoming your own watchdog.

> Conventional Wisdom:
> *Food hysteria is everywhere.*
> New Paradigm:
> *Food fraud is everywhere.*

With the terrific new FDA food labels, why should you worry? Because of food label trickery. Remember the baby food company that sold apple juice to children that was just flavored sugar water? Michael Jacobson, Ph.D., of the Center for Science in the Public

Interest says that the fraud begins with marketing to children. But even the smartest consumer can be fooled.

- Order a chef's salad only to find that the dressing has more fat than an order of french fries.
- Order lean chicken with no skin in a fruit sauce only to find that the sauce is loaded with heavy cream.
- Order a "low-fat" whole-grain muffin only to find that it contains 1,200 calories and 20 grams of fat — more than a doughnut.
- Buy low-fat yogurt only to find that it's so packed with sugar that it's classified as a carbohydrate, not a dairy product.
- Pour a bowl of cereal only to find that it has more sugar than a pack of gum.

You may mock your "granola" friends who appear to live on sprouts, whole wheat, and broccoli, but they have learned the truth: much of the nutrition has been gutted from processed foods in America. Food manufacturing and preparation leaches many of the best nutrients from foods and replaces them with cheap fillers, fats, and sugars.

If you already eat the foods described in the chapters "Multicultural Eating" and "Grazing," read no further. But if you continue to eat the traditional processed foods that line the shelves of every supermarket and convenience store in America, here's what to watch for every foot of the way to the checkout counter.

My mother is a pretty smart shopper. She came home one day with stone-ground wheat crackers from one of the major food companies. "See," she said, "we're eating healthy, too!" I looked at the label. The lead ingredients were enriched wheat flour, partially hydrogenated fat, and corn syrup. I told my mother, only half kidding, that she'd be better off buying poison. I went to the local health food store and bought her Hain Pure Foods Whole Wheat Crackers. Here the lead ingredient was organically grown stone-ground whole wheat flour. There were no fats or added sugars. In a blind taste test, both of my parents rated the second product higher. My mother said, sure, but isn't the health food brand more expensive? No way! The big food company's crackers cost $2.59 a box. Hain's cost $1.79. My mother said, "I'm sold."

WATCH OUT FOR THE BIG THREE

For more and more Americans who eat processed foods, corn syrup, white flour, and hydrogenated oils have become main staples of the American diet. It's my own opinion that many men remain fatter around the middle because they eat massive quantities of these three ingredients, all the while believing they've made good food choices just because the foods weren't loaded with saturated fats. Why are these ingredients so terrible? Inherently they bring nothing to the table except empty calories, while they replace good whole foods. As a test, go to any convenience store or grocery store. Look at the labels on crackers, bread, cereal, or snack products. I think you'll be astounded at the number of products whose chief ingredients are white flour, corn syrup, and hydrogenated oils. This is the cheapest way to make most processed foods taste good. It takes little wizardry to throw them into a box and market them.

Food labels list ingredients from the largest to the smallest amount. The labels are pretty cleverly written. The new stunt is to call white flour "wheat flour" in the hope that you will believe you are buying a whole wheat product. You're not. In parentheses, after "wheat flour," you will see a long list of vitamins, which costs food companies just pennies to include in a product and leads consumers to believe that these are the second most plentiful ingredient in the product. Many men read no further. However, at the end of the parentheses you'll see "corn syrup" and "hydrogenated oils." Here's the lowdown on the big three of processed foods.

Corn Syrup

The Department of Agriculture's Economic Research Service Report shows that Americans now eat 51.7 pounds of high-fructose corn syrup a year. That's over 25 pounds more than a decade ago.

Many men don't realize that corn syrup is in a huge number of products, from breads, crackers, and cereals to sodas and even tomato sauces. The fact remains that most of the "sugar" we eat is corn syrup. Manufacturers have switched to corn syrup because it's much cheaper than sugar or any other sweetener like honey or molasses. When I checked last summer, Midwest corn syrup cost 23½ cents a pound whereas Midwest beet sugar cost 28 cents per pound. Food companies win twice here. They get to use a cheaper product and the unsophisticated label reader thinks there's no sugar in the product. In fact the average consumer believes that corn syrup is somehow better than sugar because it's made from corn. Corn syrup can be more damaging than sugar only because of how much we eat. Corn syrup's main advantage is only for people with diabetes, because it does not increase blood sugar as much as glucose.

White Flour (Enriched Flour or Wheat Flour)

If you're trying to avoid too much sugar, corn syrup isn't the only problem. Nutritional scientist Dr. Luke Bucci says, "The body handles white flour like sugar by digesting it very quickly. Basically it's sugar strung into chains." Eating pure white-flour products is like mainlining sugar. Dr. Judith Hallfrisch of the USDA says, "White flour is very efficiently absorbed. White bread is used as the base for the Glycemic Index by Jenkins. So really it's not much different than glucose. The more fiber you eat (from whole grains), the less efficiently your gut absorbs nutrients and calories. If you eat a lot of whole foods, it decreases efficiency so less is absorbed, and you get a decrease in the actual calories you get. A lot of people get their carbohydrates from white flour, and that's bad because they should be getting it from fruits and vegetables — it would solve a lot of problems."

Chris Kilham spent years working for Whole Foods Market, one of the best health food store chains in the country. He went on to write *The Bread & Circus Whole Food Bible* and said the following: "Most cylinder and hammer mills are used to transform whole nutritious grains into nutritionally devoid white flour. In the milling process, the bran and germ layers of the grains are stripped away, leaving only the white, pulpy interior kernel, or endosperm. When whole wheat is milled into white flour, as much as 83 percent of the nutrients are removed, with mostly starch remaining. The fiber is gone, and the vitamin E content is reduced, along with 21 other nutrients. The flour that is produced is so useless as a food that it must be fortified with synthetically manufactured thiamin, riboflavin, niacin, and iron. Thirty-five of the fifty U.S. states require that white flour be thus enriched to be sold. White flour is also adulterated with chemicals used to age, bleach, whiten, and preserve the product." Even though refined white flour is widely used in baking today, this author calls white flour a "nonfood."

Critics believe that food companies use white flour because it's so cheap. White flour costs $9.58 per hundred pounds while whole wheat flour costs $10.52 per hundred pounds. White flour is found in many brands of the foods that men consider healthiest, such as bagels, pastas, breads, and cereals. If you are having trouble losing unwanted fat, consider that, in my own case, I dropped the massive amount of pasta, bagels, and bread I ate as part of a "healthy" diet and lost ten pounds in about two weeks. By eating whole grains I killed my hunger, steadied my blood sugar, and shed the extra pounds.

Hydrogenated Oils

The brunt of the coronary artery disease epidemic is traced to the second decade of this century. Some think it no accident that the first hydrogenated oil made its appearance in 1911, coinciding with the onslaught of the heart disease epidemic. To make hydrogenated fats, food manufacturers start with "good" or unsaturated fats. They then hydrogenate the liquid fat so it becomes a semi-solid. That makes the fat easier to handle and provides texture to foods. For example, it makes potato chips stay fresh and crispy. Recently the USDA released a report demonstrating that hydrogenated oils can increase cholesterol levels like the saturated fats found in hamburgers. You'll find these hydrogenated oils in most bakery items, breads, cereals, and processed foods. Food companies save about $2.00 a pound by using hydrogenated soybean oil rather than liquid canola oil. Instead of hydrogenated oils, expeller-expressed oils add none of the risk of saturated fats and all the benefits of unsaturated fats, because they are not hydrogenated. When you buy baked or processed foods, try to avoid products with labels that contain the words "hydrogenated" or "partially hydrogenated." Harvard's Dr. Walter Willett believes that these trans fatty acids, on a gram-for-gram basis, may be two to three times more dangerous than saturated fats.

READING THE LABELS

Here are some of the labeling "tricks" that even the most conscientious label readers miss. The Center for Science in the Public Interest helped me develop this list. These are all claims that slip through the labeling loopholes of the new FDA regulations. I asked Dr. Michael Jacobson of CSPI why there were so many misleading claims. "Profit" was the answer. To cut down on costs, manufacturers replace real fruit, real food, real nutrients with artificial flavoring and coloring. This cheats people out of basic nutrients.

Made with Whole Wheat

Some whole wheat crackers and whole wheat snacks are made with more white flour and oil than whole wheat flour, charges the CSPI. The labels read "wheat flour" as the lead ingredient. Whole wheat is listed, but much lower on the list. For example, graham crackers have much more white flour than graham or whole wheat flour. If you look at Teddy Grahams, they have one-fourteenth of an ounce of graham flour per one-ounce serving. CSPI has actually petitioned the FDA to ban the word "whole wheat" or "graham" from the name of any product that isn't made predominantly with whole wheat flour, since graham flour is a synonym for whole wheat.

Fruit-Juice-Sweetened

Fruit-juice-sweetened food is often the same as a food that uses white sugar or corn syrup, claims CSPI. These juices usually have been stripped of flavor and color. They have only tiny amounts of vitamins or minerals. Fruit sweeteners are boiled-down fruit. Manufacturers boil it down until there's only sugar. What you get is a combination of glucose, fructose, and sucrose. It's a syrup that's referred to as "concentrate." These products may be labeled "no sugar." Stripped juices are little more than sugar water. If you look at the first ingredient on peach fruit juice, you find that it's grape juice concentrate. In *Nutrition Action Healthletter,* Jim Tillotson, Ph.D., director of the Food Policy Institute at Tufts University, gave this advice: "In the supermarket, if I saw white grape, apple, or pear juice concentrate, I'd be suspicious." According to nutrition scientist Luke Bucci, Ph.D., of SpectraCell Labs in Houston, fruit sweeteners are not any better than table sugar. Many health food products use fruit juice sweeteners to make them appear healthy. I've found that these products often have a very peculiar flavor. My least favorite are cereals sweetened with pear juice. I'd much rather have the cereal unsweetened and add a teaspoon of honey or table sugar. These natural products are competing with major cereal companies who often use corn syrup to sweeten even "unsweetened" cereals like cornflakes.

Made with Real Fruit

Here's the same problem in a different disguise. These products use white grape juice sweeteners, grape juice concentrate, and other stripped sugars. The fruit they have is in near trace amounts. One children's snack has one-seventeenth of an orange. Another company's cereal bar has one-fiftieth of an apple.

Modified Food Starch

These are thickening agents that replace much more expensive and nutritious ingredients.

Enriched Flour

CSPI would like to see "enriched flour" renamed "partially restored flour." Once flour is milled, it is usually stripped of the germ and bran layers, which contain a wealth of fiber, vitamins, and minerals.

Some B vitamins and iron are added back, but it's a far cry from whole grain.

Fortified Cereals

When you buy a cereal fortified with masses of vitamins, you're usually getting sprayed-on vitamins. David Schardt of CSPI says, "There's not a lot of information available. The cereal companies won't talk to you about it. However, spraying, with a vitamin mixture, is the most common way to fortify flakes. The one potential problem that we do know about is that the nutrients don't last forever. This depends on the conditions under which the cereal is maintained. The hotter and more humid something is, the more exposed to the air, the shorter the lifetime of the nutrients. These nutrients are the same as you would find in a vitamin pill."

The point is this: why not eat cereals that have naturally occurring vitamins contained in whole grains?

Chicken

Unless the ingredients on chicken nuggets or chicken breast patties read "chicken meat," there's probably chicken skin in the product. Misleading labels may read "chicken breast," "chicken thigh," or just plain "chicken." Patties and nuggets are usually breaded. Up to 30 percent of the total weight may be breading.

The new FDA label doesn't flag trans fatty acids, nor does it tip you off to the amount of white flour or corn syrup, but it's still a valuable tool. Commissioner David Kessler told me first to concentrate on the total fat, cholesterol, and sodium stated on the label. None should exceed 5 percent in healthy foods. Next look for sugars. The label doesn't distinguish between refined and naturally occurring sugars. Five grams is a reasonable amount for healthy cereals and baked products. Then read the ingredients list. For grain products, the first ingredients should be oat bran, whole wheat, oats, or other whole grains, instead of wheat flour or enriched flour. Scan the rest of the list for hydrogenated or partially hydrogenated oils or corn syrup.

The bottom line is that your intake of refined sugars should be 10 percent or less of your diet. The average American diet is made up of 20 percent simple sugars. Misleading labels can push that up to 30 percent or more for men trying to eat less and less fat by eating more and more carbos without checking the label first.

Chapter 11

Sports Foods

IT'S 6:50 A.M. YOUR HEART IS THUMPING A MERE THIRTY-EIGHT BEATS A minute. With the alarm, you roll out of bed onto a single bent knee. Like a freshly pummeled prizefighter, you slowly and carefully rise through a foglike trance and stumble into the kitchen. Like a drug addict fumbling for a badly needed fix you mix 660 calories of dynamite-packed protein powder and power-blaster carbohydrate with ice and water. The life-giving potion stirs in the blender on high-speed crush control. The blender spins down. You gulp down a full quart in seconds. Wham! You're back!

Few concepts are more alluring than special foods that can transform a man's performance into that of a stronger, faster, more powerful athlete. Unfortunately, most weekend warriors practice very primitive forms of fueling. Even Olympic athletes are more likely to hurt their performance than help due to an unsophisticated knowledge of sports nutrition. Why? Fueling high-performance exercise is more complex than mixing rocket fuels and is fraught with easily made errors. To fill this void, industry has come up with a whole new kind of food to make fueling for exercise simpler and more efficient. They succeeded in creating sports foods that have become a hot commodity in bike shops, health food stores, and camping outfitters. Unfortunately, many sports foods are 50 percent hype, 40 percent marketing, and only 10 percent nutrition. The race is so fast and furious to get into this business that little thought goes into many of these products. The most popular are power bars, sports drinks, and protein powders.

Conventional Wisdom:
Grab a Coke.
New Paradigm:
Grab a power bar.

I have not run into a single man over thirty-five who doesn't take some special performance-enhancing potion. At McCarthy's, the breakfast hangout in Stowe, Vermont, a logger explained how brewer's yeast kept him young. Mike Farney, a long-time cross-country skiing friend, sold me on using Klamath Lakes Super Blue Green Algae. Charles H. Hennekens, M.D., a professor at Harvard Medical School, takes vitamin E as part of an ongoing study to prevent cardiovascular disease. Austin Hearst, a television executive, takes dozens of supplements to improve his rock climbing, with remarkable success. The trouble is that every man takes something entirely different and yet swears that only his special supplement really works. Here's what the scientists say works best.

STRATEGIES

1. Reload Muscle Fuel Stores Quickly

Reloading muscle fuel stores is the best and most practical application of sports fuels. The bad news is that muscle fuel stores are the hardest and slowest to fill yet are the most critical for virtually every kind of exercise. The better stocked your muscles are with fuel, the faster and farther you can go. Right after a workout there is a small window of opportunity during which you can have a dramatic effect on your recovery. The right fuels will refill your muscles faster and more completely than is possible at any other time. Dr. John Ivy's breakthrough research at the University of Texas at Austin demonstrates that the addition of protein to carbohydrate speeds the refilling of muscle sugar stores. The ratio he recommends is 2.5 grams of carbohydrate to 1 gram of protein. A 200-pound man would take 100 grams of carbohydrate with 40 grams of protein immediately after exercise and again two hours later. Dr. Ivy used a test product from Shaklee called Yamanouchi Physique in his research. I mix my own, using three scoops of Opti Fuel 2 with one scoop of Nitro Fuel or pure whey protein.

Here's why it works. The combination of animal protein and fast-burning sugars raises insulin to very high levels. High insulin levels effect the fastest, most complete refilling of muscle sugar stores. Research confirms that reloading with fast-burning sugars is more effective than slow-burning carbos. Specially formulated sports drinks contain these simple sugars in concentrations that you can easily absorb. If you prefer foods, you can eat fast-burning, easily digestible carbohydrates such as sweet potatoes. The one simple sugar that won't help much in reloading your muscle is fructose. If downing a sugary sports drink after exercise pops your blood sugar into low earth orbit, here's some advice. Remember, right after exercise your muscles crave sugar and suck it up like a sponge. My best experience has been to get slow-burning carbos into my system about forty-five minutes after the last dose of fast-burning carbos so that I dampen the drop in blood sugar. It's like putting nice slow-burning logs into a fireplace just after you've thrown in the Sunday paper. For everyday use, take only the immediate post-exercise dose and skip the second one because of the high number of calories. It still works pretty well. Here are several other theoretical advantages to reloading with a protein-carbohydrate beverage.

- You supply muscles with protein when it's needed the most. Carbohydrates with protein refuel muscles faster than any other means possible. The influx of amino acids into muscles is thought to be greatest at the end of exercise. Carbohydrates and protein cause a surge of insulin that may allow great quantities of amino acids to flood into the muscles.

- You increase muscle-building hormones. Dr. John Ivy's research suggests that human growth hormone levels are increased and more testosterone is made available to muscles. Both of these hormones have strong muscle-building properties.
- Since amino acids circulate for only three hours after consumption, it makes sense to take them when your body can use them most. If you want to do with less protein, you can consider concentrating it around your workouts, when it will do the most good, and cutting back for other meals.

This technique is still considered experimental and should be avoided by anyone with diabetes or a history of low blood sugar.

2. Keep Muscles Well Fueled

Research shows that fueling before exercise improves both the endurance and the intensity of exercise. That can be accomplished with foods well before exercise or sports fuels immediately before.

Pre-exercise food. The pretraining meal has a very simple purpose: to make certain that muscle and liver fuel tanks are topped off. This meal can't make up for poor nutrition or for failure to refuel immediately after exercise as described above. If your muscle fuel tanks are half full, this meal won't do much. However, it can top off liver fuel stores, which are critical to maintaining steady blood sugar levels during sustained exercise.

Be warned that eating before exercise should be carefully planned, since it often does more harm than good. Taken too soon before exercise, the meal can cause your blood sugar to soar and then crash once exercise begins. If your stomach has not completely emptied, you will have gastric acid, food, and fluid sloshing around as you work out. To avoid a crashing blood sugar level or slop in your stomach, most nutritionists recommend a meal four hours before training or competition. The composition of that meal is critical. It should be largely slow-burning carbohydrates with some protein and little fat. The protein will curb your hunger as will the slow-burning carbos so that you won't be as tempted to eat closer to training. Fats take up to eight hours to digest, so they sit in your intestine during exercise. A large reservoir of any food in your intestine does you no good, since so little of it can be digested during exercise. The unused portion is just dead weight that can suck water out of the blood-stream into the intestine. The four-hour time limit allows blood sugar levels to return to normal and much of your last meal to clear from your stomach.

Pre-exercise sports drinks. Sports foods are used when there is no time to digest a meal, typically ten minutes before exercise begins. There are several theoretical advantages to a pretraining sports fuel before prolonged exercise. The most prominent are to prevent a large drop in blood volume once exercise begins and to enhance performance. I also like a pretraining beverage, because I think it makes my brain more favorably disposed to working out. Be warned that this is the trickiest time to use sports fuels, and it is unnecessary if you've had a good meal four hours before.

Since real food does such a good job of topping off your fuel tanks before exercise, the most practical reason for taking a sports drink is when you work out first thing in the morning. Blood sugar levels are low, around 70, and will take a long time to rise during exercise without any added fuel. In fact, after an overnight fast, your liver fuel stores may be nearly empty and your blood sugar may actually fall further with exercise! If you're already at 70 or 80 and you exercise for a long period of time, it can drop to 50 or 60, which can be quite detrimental to performance.

Dr. Keith Wheeler, of Ross Laboratories in Columbus, Ohio, says, "If you fast an individual for 12 to 14 hours and their blood sugar levels are on the lower end, about 75–80 starting out, that decreases performance by 30–40 percent." Keith does point out that there are those who can stand to train fasting and others who can't: "It truly is individual. Someone like Dave Scott, the professional endurance triathlete who has won six Iron Man contests, who has been shown to be a very extreme fat burner, he's very efficient in using fats in his body. He then takes advantage of that by training his body further to burn fat. Other people simply can't get away with it, because their body is not genetically predisposed to using fat at a very high rate." I like to load up if I'm going for a long workout at a moderate intensity. There's that much less fluid to carry with me and it gives me a psychological boost. Some research shows that pre-exercise beverages do boost your pace and endurance. Dr. W. Michael Sherman, of Ohio State University's Department of Health, Physical Education and Recreation, confirms that. "We found that, contrary to what most experts think, ingesting carbohydrates in the form of sugar-sweetened sports drinks before prolonged exercise improved performance."

Sample fuel: I'll have 100 grams of carbohydrate and 15 grams of protein in a liter of water before a two-hour morning workout. I use Opti Fuel 2 and spike it with Ripped Fuel or Hot Stuff.

3. Preserve Muscle Fuel Levels During Prolonged Exercise

The conventional wisdom is that you don't need sports fuel for intense exercise under ninety minutes, since you should have all the fuel you need stored in your muscle fuel tanks. Over the ninety-minute mark, you may preserve muscle fuel levels and keep your blood sugar up by taking sports fuels. Dr. Andrew Coggan, an exercise physiologist at the University of Texas Medical Branch in Galveston, recommends the following: "Ingest carbohydrates at a rate of 160 to 300 calories per hour throughout exercise. You'll keep your blood sugar constant and delay fatigue. Another option is to consume 200 grams late in exercise, but well before fatigue sets in. But if you wait for fatigue, refueling is pretty ineffective and you're unlikely to maintain a normal blood sugar." Studies show that both methods prevent fatigue and maintain intensity equally well. Sample fuels are Hydra Fuel from Twin Labs and Cytomax from Champion Nutrition.

The most cutting edge sports drinks contain a small amount of protein. Research by Dr. Bill Evans of Pennsylvania State University concludes that 85 to 90 percent of the body's daily supply of the amino acid leucine is consumed during a two-hour bike ride. The theory is that if you drink a beverage with protein during a workout, you're supplying muscle with leucine so that it doesn't break down. Since endurance athletes do break down muscle during intense training, research suggests that you can cut fatigue, muscle soreness, and recovery time while lifting your spirits and pumping your immune system. I've found I'm less sore after a tough endurance workout if there's protein in the recovery beverage. Several commercial preparations include protein in their carbohydrate beverages, including liquid Nitro Fuel from Twin Labs and Blue Thunder from American Body Building Products. These drinks are much more concentrated than you would want for endurance work. I dilute them with one or two equal volumes of water. Cyclists are concerned that too much protein can pull water out of the bloodstream and into the stomach and intestine. The strategy that I've adapted is to drink a beverage that has a high concentration of the amino acid leucine so that less raw protein is required.

The use of protein drinks during exercise is just in its infancy. For that reason, you're truly experimenting whenever you take them. In the next several years, you'll probably see protein used in sports drinks for shorter-duration, higher-intensity work like skiing and tennis matches. The most intriguing reason for taking protein during a workout is that it prevents mental fatigue. As your body consumes amino acids circulating in the blood and lowers their concentration, carbohydrates have much easier access to the brain. Since carbohydrates make brain chemicals that make you sleepy and protein makes brain chemicals that make you alert, it makes sense that you'll have less brain fatigue with more protein. In fact, research demonstrated an increase in IQ and alertness when protein drinks were ingested by athletes during a soccer game. For long endurance workouts or competitions, you may want to experiment with adding a little protein, no more than one gram for every five grams of carbohydrate.

Dr. John Ivy has found a really interesting application of sports fuels. If your exercise varies in intensity between moderate and vigorous, taking a sports drink may spare some of your critical muscle fuel stores. This may be a good excuse to use sports drinks during long tennis matches, for a several-hour-long ski session, or during a hike or bike ride over undulating terrain. The rationale is that you don't deplete those hard-to-fill muscle fuel tanks and you'll be able to play harder that day and the next.

Supplements taken during a workout need to be dilute enough so they don't get trapped in your stomach. Any beverage with a concentration over 8 percent empties slowly from the stomach.

Liquids have been considered better than solid foods during exercise because they are easier to ingest and don't require having a separate supply of water to wash them down. However, recent research shows that you'll go just as far just as fast with sports bars as sports drinks. In some situations sports bars have the advantage. By carrying water and sports bars you can mix and match as you choose. This is particularly convenient when exercising in the heat. You can drink pure water when you're thirsty, then eat a sports bar before your energy flags. For very long events, most athletes want real food. I know that after the first six hours of a twenty-four-hour bike race I had to have real food. However, at the lowered intensity of very long competitions, there is less urgency to be scientifically precise and more time to eat. For very high intensity workouts and races, it's much harder to eat than it is to drink. By experimenting with different concentrations in different temperatures and different intensity workouts, you'll know exactly what replacement options to have at the ready.

SPORTS BARS

At 180-plus calories, sports bars are really minimeals complete with protein, carbohydrate, fat, fiber, minerals, and vitamins. For that reason I look for the same balance and quality I would in a meal. They should contain excellent-quality milk proteins and whole-grain carbohydrates, both of which will steady your blood sugar. However, you'll find even the best bars are nearly schizophrenic in wanting to be everything from a hiker's snack to a triathlete's race fuel.

If you grew up on Baby Ruths and Twinkies, you're in for a big surprise. Most bars don't hit you between the eyes with taste or lift your spirits with the soaring sugar high of a great candy bar. First taste impressions range from yuck to the unprintable. Actual taste ranges from sawdust to a not-sweet-enough candy bar. But during exercise most athletes don't like sticky-sweet products because they don't taste healthy and use too many concentrated sugars. The best advice is to look beyond the taste to content and make your decision based on what the bar will do for you. I'm distressed by the number of sports publications that rate the bars on taste and turn a blind eye to a bar's real nutritional value. Whatever bar you choose, after a few days you won't give taste a second thought.

Sports bars should feel light in your stomach. Bars eaten during moderate-to-intense exercise should break down in the digestive tract and be absorbed quickly. Bars eaten for low-to-moderate exercise of long duration, such as hiking, should contain fiber, protein, and high-quality complex carbos to slow down absorption.

Sports bars start at 180 calories but quickly make their way up to over 600! Since the body can process only a very limited amount of food during exercise, beware of high-calorie bars. I like to stay in the 180 to 270 range.

Couldn't you just eat a candy bar? Most candy bars just sit in your stomach during exercise. Their high sugar content slows absorption from the stomach while their high fat content requires a prolonged time to digest. Good sports bars have made such a hit because they are easily absorbed, readily supply sugar to muscle and the brain, and don't have much fat.

INGREDIENTS

Slow-Burning Carbohydrates

If you are using a sports bar as a substitute meal; for low-intensity activities like hiking, golf, an afternoon of doubles tennis; or hours before high-intensity exercise, choose a bar with high-quality complex carbohydrates such as oats, bran, whole wheat, and other whole-grain ingredients that provide extra minerals, vitamins, fiber, and antioxidants. Don't mistake glucose polymers, rice dextrin, and maltodextrins for high-quality, slow-burning carbos. They are stripped of fiber and other whole-food benefits. Their advantage is only for high-intensity exercise because they enter the bloodstream quickly like simple sugars.

Fast-burning Carbohydrates

Sugars make sports bars taste slightly better than sawdust. On the label sugars are listed as sucrose, glucose, fructose, fruit juice concentrates, corn syrup, honey, or the more sophisticated maltodextrins, polyglucose, or glucose polymers. Many of the cheaper bars use corn syrup or high-fructose corn syrup as a major ingredient to make them sound high-tech and healthy. Corn syrup is the cheapest and easiest way to add carbohydrates. Glucose and glucose polymers work best only during sustained moderate to high-intensity exercise. Look for them on the label. Here's where the schizophrenic approach lies. Most manufacturers dump in lots of fast-burning carbos to make the product look like a high-performance bar or to make it taste sweet. However, they then add slow-burning carbos to play it safe and make the bar look healthy. As a result most bars are neither a pure fast-burning carbo bar for intense exercise nor a slow-burning carbo bar for low-intensity exercise or snacking. Manufacturers try to get around this inconsistency by promoting the slow, steady release of sugars that the combination of fast and slow sugars provides. I don't buy it.

Fructose. There's no good evidence that fructose makes you go faster or farther. Fructose cannot be as readily absorbed and used by muscle as glucose, since it must first go to the liver to be processed. A small amount of fructose in a sports drink can help gastric emptying and refuel the liver during exercise, neither of which makes much of a real difference in increased speed or endurance. You should avoid bars with more than 10 percent fructose during exercise, since they can cause nausea and diarrhea. Even the best bars have masses of fructose, which seems pointless to me. The rationale is that the bar tastes sweet but doesn't create a fast rise and fall of blood sugar. Good-quality complex carbos like oats and brans would steady blood sugar and impart much greater food value. If you're using a bar for high performance and need simple sugars, glucose and glucose polymers are far more effective and lack the side effects of fructose. Many manufacturers fear the bars won't be used for intense exercise and so rightly omit the glucose but, unfortunately, bypass the grains.

Natural juice sweeteners. Fruit sweeteners are boiled-down fruit. Manufacturers boil it until there's only sugar. What you get is a combination of glucose, fructose, and sucrose. It's a syrup that's referred to as "concentrate." "Natural juice sweeteners" on the label makes the product sound superhealthy when it's really not.

Protein

Protein makes up 10 to 30 percent of total calories in high-quality sports bars. During exercise you don't need more than 15 percent if the protein is high quality, such as milk proteins or whey. Many bars have incomplete proteins that do nothing to improve performance. Look for high-quality milk proteins like whey.

Fat

Fats are used to make the bar stick together or make it taste better. Anything over three grams isn't really necessary. Most high-quality bars do without any fat.

Fiber

Large amounts of fiber are not necessary in sports bars during high-intensity training, because fiber takes up room needed for other, more important ingredients and slows absorption. As a meal or for low-intensity long-duration events, fiber helps to keep blood sugar at a nice even level. If you're using these bars as meal substitutes, look for a high fiber content.

Supplements

Bars contain everything from selenium and chromium to molybdenum and ginseng. While there are good theoretical reasons for all of them, first-class controlled trials are sorely lacking. One popular example is carnitine, which makes a lot of sense, theoretically. However, a recent study by Dr. David Costill, director of the Human Performance Lab at Ball State University in Muncie, Indiana, shows that the muscle just doesn't need any more than it already has. If you make a decision to take supplements, buy them individually rather than in a shotgun blast from a sports bar. You're far more certain of getting the quality and quantity you want.

The following products illustrate what to look for on the label of a sports bar. The more fast-burning carbos, the better the bar is for intense exercise. The more slow-burning carbos, the better the bar is for low-intensity exercise and for use as a minimeal.

PowerBar
Powerfood Inc.

This is the most famous sports bar of all. Available in Malt Nut, Banana, Mocha, Chocolate, Apple Cinnamon, and Wildberry; one bar contains 225 calories, 2 grams of fat, 3 grams of fiber, and 90 mg of sodium.

Pro:
- Soluble fibers from oat bran replace fat.
- Excellent protein:
  — 10 grams of high-quality lactose-free, total milk protein with a good amino acid profile.
  — 200 mg of free-form amino acids such as leucine, valine, and isoleucine.
- 100 percent of the RDA of vitamins C, E, B_1, B_2, B_3, B_5, B_6, and B_{12}.

Con:
- 15 grams of fructose from grape, corn, and pear sources.

Performance-related data:
Cyclists who ingested the PowerBar five minutes prior to cycling rode longer to fatigue: 57.4 minutes, compared to the placebo group, which rode to 42.9 minutes.

FAST-BURNING CARBOS: maltodextrins.

SLOW-BURNING CARBOS: oat bran, brown rice.

Clif Bar
Kali's Bakery
Available in five flavors — Apricot, Apple/Cherry, Fig/Raisin, Dark Chocolate, and Crunchy Chocolate Chip — Clif Bars contain whole grains, fruit, and natural sweeteners, not highly processed ingredients. These bars are baked, not extruded. One bar has 245 calories, 2 grams of fat, 3 grams of fiber, and 20 to 100 mg of sodium, depending on the flavor.

Pro:
• Great whole-food product.
• Baked bar is easier to digest.

Con:
• Too much fructose: 16 grams of simple sugars from fruit and grape juice concentrate.
• Low in protein:
  — Only 5 grams.
  — Protein comes from oats, which is an incomplete protein.
• Some flavors have high sodium levels.

Performance-related data:
FAST-BURNING CARBOS: none.

SLOW-BURNING CARBOS: rolled oats, cornmeal, oat bran.

Forza
Universal Labs
Available in Vanilla Malt, Chocolate, Veryberry, and Applepie; one bar contains 233 calories, 1 gram of fat, 4 grams of fiber, and 65 mg of sodium.

Pro:
• 11 grams of high-quality protein from milk and soy.

Performance-related data:
FAST-BURNING CARBOS: maltodextrins, honey, raisins.

SLOW-BURNING CARBOS: oat bran, brown rice.

Exceed Sports Bar

Weider Food Companies

Available in Banana, Chocolate, and Oatbran; one bar contains 280 calories, 2 grams of fat, 3 grams of fiber, and 150 mg of sodium.

Pro:

• 13 grams of protein from milk-protein concentrate.

Con:

• High in sodium.

• 26 grams of high-fructose corn syrup.

Performance-related data:

FAST-BURNING CARBOS: sucrose, glucose polymers.

SLOW-BURNING CARBOS: oat bran.

Edgebar

Nutritional N-ER-G Products, Inc.

Available in Citrus, Chocolate, and Vanilla; one bar contains 240 calories, less than 2 grams of fat, 2.5 grams of fiber, and 60 mg of sodium.

Pro:

• 10 grams of whey protein.

Con:

• 23 grams of fructose.

Performance-related data:

FAST-BURNING CARBOS: maltodextrins.

SLOW-BURNING CARBOS: 23 grams from bran and puffed brown rice.

New Ultra Fuel

Twin Labs

Available in Chocolate, Vanilla, Banana, and Berry; one bar contains 260 calories, no fat, 2 grams of fiber, and 40 mg of sodium.

Pro:

• 15 grams of high-quality protein from whey and calcium caseinate.

• Fat-free.

Con:
- 12.5 grams of simple carbohydrate from fructose.

Performance-related data:
Only bar with a high amount of fast-burning sugars for high-intensity workouts.

FAST-BURNING CARBOS: 37.5 grams of maltodextrins.
SLOW-BURNING CARBOS: none.

Diet Fuel
Twin Labs
Available in Chocolate, Vanilla, Banana, and Berry; one bar contains 180 calories, no fat, 5 grams of fiber, and 10 mg of sodium.

Pro:
- 15 grams of high-quality protein from whey and calcium caseinate.

Con:
- 14 grams of crystalline pure fructose as the first ingredient.

Performance-related data:
FAST-BURNING CARBOS: none.
SLOW-BURNING CARBOS: polydextrose.

Parrillo
Parrillo Performance
Available in Chocolate, Vanilla, Peanut Butter, Layered Peanut Butter Chocolate; one bar contains 240 calories, 1 gram of fat, 2 grams of fiber, and 50 mg of sodium.

Pro:
- No high-fructose corn syrup.
- 11 grams of quality protein from calcium caseinate, hydrolyzed lactalbumin, and potassium lactalbumin.
- 5.5 grams of the medium-chained fatty acid CapTri.

Con:
- Some nutritionists say that MCT (medium-chained triglycerides) oil is just an ordinary fat. John Parrillo and many top athletes believe that MCT is a high-performance fat. Most academics disagree.

127

Performance-related data:
FAST-BURNING CARBOS: rice dextrin, maltodextrin.
SLOW-BURNING CARBOS: oat bran, brown rice, rice bran.

BTU Stoker

BTU Stoker, Inc.
Available in Cocoa and Apple/Oat; one bar contains 252 calories, 3 grams of fat, 3.9 grams of fiber, and 21 mg of sodium.

Pro:
• No high-fructose corn syrup.
• 3.9 grams of fiber.
• 10 grams of protein from calcium caseinate.
• Good whole-food ingredients.

Performance-related data:
FAST-BURNING CARBOS: rice dextrin plus 15 percent simple sugars, maltodextrin, raisins.
SLOW-BURNING CARBOS: oat bran, crisped rice, rice bran, apples.

Hot Stuff

National Health Products
Available only in Pineapple; one bar contains 270 calories, 2 grams of fat, 2 grams of fiber, and 35 mg of sodium.

Pro:
• 15 grams of quality protein from calcium caseinate, whey, protein concentrate, and toasted rolled oats.

Con:
• 20 grams of high-fructose corn syrup.

Performance-related data:
FAST-BURNING CARBOS: glucose polymers, honey.
SLOW-BURNING CARBOS: 26 grams from toasted rolled oats, crisped rice.

finHälsa

finHälsa Company

Most bars have a carbohydrate-to-protein ratio of 4 to 1. Finhälsa has a 2.5 to 1 ratio. Available in Raisin Nut Crunch and Raspberry Crunch; one bar contains 170 calories, 2 grams of fat, 4 grams of fiber, and 98 mg of sodium.

Pro:

- Protein acts as a chaser behind the carb to stabilize blood glucose levels longer. You won't get a spike in insulin response.
- 11 grams of protein from calcium sodium caseinate.

Con:

- 4 grams of fructose syrup, which is the first ingredient.

Performance-related data:

FAST-BURNING CARBOS: maltodextrins.

SLOW-BURNING CARBOS: wheat germ nuggets, raisins, soy concentrate, oat bran, and barley malt.

SPORTS DRINKS

Sports drinks are nearly a billion-dollar industry. Since most sports scientists say sports drinks won't enhance performance for workouts and races longer than ninety minutes, why have they become so popular with men who do much less exercise or none at all? The sports drinks' biggest plus is in the rehydration arena. Most men are simply willing to drink more of a slightly sweetened drink than they are water, since thirst is not a strong enough stimulus to get people to drink enough in hot weather.

It's best to chill these drinks. Cold beverages empty from the stomach faster than warm ones. Cold beverages rate much higher in palatability. Both of these factors add up to more fluid intake if a beverage is cold.

A highly sophisticated study traced specially tagged water molecules from the stomach into the bloodstream. The result? An 8 percent solution was in the bloodstream faster than a 2.5 percent solution during intense prolonged exercise. Most commercially available drinks fall in the 4 to 8 percent sugar range. Concentrations higher than 8 percent don't empty from the stomach as quickly.

Everyone can benefit from ingesting 240 to 280 calories per hour during exercise that's longer than ninety minutes. Try eight ounces every twenty minutes of an 8 percent solution. Why not just down a soft drink or fruit juice? Soft drinks and concentrated fruit juices can cause abdominal cramps and nausea. Sodas or fruit juices also pass slowly from the stomach to the small intestine.

INGREDIENTS

Glucose Polymers

High-tech manufacturers use glucose polymers, which are long chains of sugar molecules conventionally listed on food and beverage labels as maltodextrins. The theory is that large numbers of individual sugar molecules stay in the stomach longer, but if linked together, they would leave the stomach faster. However, experiments by Dr. David Costill showed that polymers don't leave the stomach any faster than individual sugar molecules. Their theoretical advantage is that they deliver more fuel into your intestine without slowing up the delivery from the stomach. While that's a great idea, the studies that have been done show that there really is no difference between a glucose polymer and a simple sugar in terms of performance. There is one practical advantage. Glucose polymers aren't as sweet, so that you are likely to drink more fluid. The high-tech aspect of these drinks really boils down to palatability. Glucose polymers are better than simple sugars in their ability to allow rapid hydration during exercise even with the carbohydrate.

Protein

Sports drinks with protein are just beginning to emerge on the market. Since protein fuels 15 percent of exercise, the rationale is that you won't break down muscle if you feed protein. Early complaints about protein drinks came from cyclists who said that the protein tended to suck water into their stomachs, making them feel uncomfortable. I think the future of protein in sports drinks is to use small quantities of very high still quality protein. Since it is the branched-chain amino acid leucine that's most in demand, sports drinks with leucine may prevent fatigue and muscle breakdown. Ingredient labels that list branched-chain amino acids (such as isoleucine and leucine) or whey protein from blue-chip manufacturers are what I look for.

Minerals

It's not unreasonable to have a small quantity in a sports beverage for very long workouts, but for shorter periods, your best bet is to replenish these minerals and salts with your next meal. Concentrated solutions of minerals and salts just aren't necessary and can be dangerous since they can cause high concentrates in the blood.

Virtually all of the following products are formulated with fast-burning sugars for prolonged, high-intensity workouts.

Nitro Fuel
Twin Labs

Available in Natural Orange, Fruit Punch, Grape; each serving contains 460 calories and no fat. The addition of a small amount of high-quality protein makes this the prototype drink of the future.

Pro:
- 15 grams of super-high-quality ion-exchange whey protein.
- Contains chromium picolinate and alpha ketoglutarate.
- Studies indicate that dietary protein/amino acid needs may be increased by regular high-intensity exercise training. According to Steve Blechman, vice president of new product development and marketing at Twin Labs, Nitro Fuel contains "the ultimate anti-catabolic combination of protein/amino acids and carbohydrates which is crucial for nitrogen retention and muscle tissue repair."

Con:
- 25 grams of crystalline fructose.
- Very concentrated; needs to be diluted.

Hydra Fuel

Twin Labs

Available in Natural Orange, Lemon-Lime, Fruit Punch, and Grape; each serving contains 132 calories and no fat.

Pro:

- 23 grams of fast carbos from glucose polymers and glucose.
- Replenishes important electrolytes: sodium, potassium, magnesium, and chloride.
- Performance studies indicate that Hydra Fuel's 7 percent carbohydrate content is optimum for fluid replacement and energy during prolonged physical activity. Its combination of glucose and sodium has proven most effective for promoting rapid fluid absorption and preventing dehydration.

Con:

- 10 grams simple carbohydrate from fructose — a small amount, says Twin Labs, to enhance gastric emptying.

Ultra Fuel

Twin Labs

Available in Natural Orange, Grape, Lemon-Lime, Fruit Punch, and Grape; each serving contains 400 calories and no fat.

Pro:

- 75 grams of fast carbos from maltodextrins.
- Provides chromium, potassium, magnesium, phosphate, B complex vitamins, and 100 percent of the RDA for vitamin C.

Con:

- 25 grams of simple carbohydrate from pure crystalline fructose.
- A lot of calories; needs to be diluted.

Neosource Colgan Institute Meal Replacement Protein Shake

Neogen

Available in Chocolate and Strawberry/Banana; each serving contains 122 calories and 1 gram of fat with 0 percent saturated fat.

Pro:

- 5 grams of fast carbos from maltodextrins.
- 17 grams of protein from whey and egg white.
- 4 grams of dietary fiber.

Con:

- 11 grams of fructose.

Shaklee Performance Maximum Endurance Sports Drink

Shaklee Corporation

This drink was originally designed to fuel a pilot-pedaled plane featured in *National Geographic*. The drink needed to be concentrated enough to provide adequate carbohydrate fuel to peddle the seventy-two miles from Crete to Santorini in the Greek Islands. Available in Orange and Lemon-Lime; each serving contains 100 calories and no fat. Shaklee will not release specific information on the grams of simple and complex carbs.

Pro:

- Electrolytes such as potassium, calcium, sodium, phosphorous, chloride, and magnesium.
- Performance-related data shows that cyclists who ingested Shaklee increased their endurance. After they cycled at variable intensities for a few hours, researchers significantly increased intensity on cyclists who ingested Shaklee and cyclists who ingested the placebo. Cyclists who ingested Shaklee were able to continue exercising for thirty-three minutes, while the placebo group continued to exercise for only two minutes.

Exceed Energy Drink

Weider Food Companies

Available in Lemon-Lime and Orange; each serving contains 70 calories and no fat.

Pro:

- Performance-related testing in triathletes by Dr. Mindy Millard-Stafford at Georgia Institute of Technology demonstrated that consuming Exceed over plain water during simulated triathlons improved performance significantly. Exceed shortened time by 15 percent and therefore improved performance.

• Contains electrolytes: sodium, potassium, calcium, and magnesium.

Con:
• 7 grams of fructose.

PowerAde
The Coca-Cola Company
This sports drink is a fluid-replacement drink. Available in Lemon-Lime, Orange, Fruit Punch, and Grape; each serving contains 70 calories and no fat.

Pro:
• Added electrolytes.
• Georgia Tech's Dr. Mindy Millard-Stafford recently completed a study that compared PowerAde, Gatorade, and water. Highly trained male runners were asked to run about eight miles and then to run a ninth mile all out. An hour before running, each runner drank one liter of either PowerAde, Gatorade, or water. In the ninth mile, the runners who consumed PowerAde ran 17 seconds faster and those who drank Gatorade ran 14 seconds faster than those who drank the water.

Con:
• High-fructose corn syrup is the second ingredient.
• No protein.

Gatorade
The Gatorade Company
This drink comes in eight different flavors; each serving contains 50 calories and no fat.

Pro:
• Added electrolytes for superhydration and increased energy needed to help improve performance.
• Dr. Ed Coyle, director of the Human Performance Lab, Department

of Kinesiology and Health Education at the University of Texas at Austin, has conducted studies showing Gatorade to enhance endurance performance when consumed during long-duration exercises. Gatorade has been compared to water, and you can go longer with the Gatorade.

Con:

• No protein.

PROTEIN POWDERS

First-of-its-kind research shows that novice bodybuilders and serious endurance athletes have an increased protein requirement, which appears to be well above the recommended daily allowance. Those amounts are listed in Chapter 6, "Get Hard." While men can and do get that protein from real food, protein powders are now entering the mainstream of fitness from the netherworld of bodybuilding. Here are the key selling points put forward by researchers and industry.

• High-quality protein supplements have zero percent fat.
• Muscle soreness at the end of exercise may occur because muscle has been used as a fuel during prolonged exercise. By adding branched-chain amino acids to replacement fluids, less breakdown may occur, since key BCAAs are consumed in the greatest quantity during exercise.
• When students at Old Dominion University in Norfolk, Virginia, simulated a triathlon, those taking BCAAs ran a minute per mile faster than those who didn't.
• Protein taken with carbohydrate at the end of exercise helps to refuel muscle fuel tanks much faster than carbohydrate alone. Extra protein helps store much more carbohydrate than would otherwise be possible. Recovery is faster.
• Exercise lowers the body's level of an amino acid called glutamine. Lower glutamine levels may help explain the suppression in immune response seen in athletes training heavily. Swim team members at Old Dominion University who took glutamine had improved immune response and less overtraining.

• New muscle is just plain harder to build as you get older. Researchers are probing the use of protein powders to build muscle for senior citizens. Industry claims that BCAAs and other special ingredients may have special muscle-building properties.

I'd be misleading you if I told you that taking protein supplements was not controversial. I've personally found them to be very helpful but feel that you should hear both sides of the story. Here's what the critics say.

• You get all the protein you need in a balanced diet. Individual amino acids are dangerous. Most supplements are whole-protein products concentrated from milk, eggs, and other foods. However, some products advertise that they add high concentrations of individual amino acids. The FDA thinks that they're dangerous. In 1993 the FDA released a report suggesting that the consumption of individual amino acids may be quite harmful, although it had no convincing proof.

• Excess protein is bad for you. Once you consume over 200 grams of protein a day, you may be in trouble. High levels of protein intake result in high levels of ammonia and urea in your blood. A perfectly healthy young person can overload his kidneys' ability to dump these compounds. The result is a feeling of fatigue and pain in the lower back. Excess protein can also wash calcium out of bone, creating early osteoporosis.

• Protein powders contain too much sugar. If you've never tasted the powders that come in the big tubs at health food stores, try some. You'll immediately notice that some are almost sickeningly sweet. Why? First, they have to disguise the otherwise disgusting taste of ingredients like predigested beef glands. Second, they need enough carbohydrate with them to drive up insulin to get the protein into muscle cells. Richard Wurtman, M.D., a professor of neuroscience and the director of the Clinical Research Center at MIT, says that 50 grams is all the carbohydrate you need to push protein into muscle. The best protein powders use high-quality whey that doesn't require any disguising. You can add your own carbohydrate to it.

INGREDIENTS

If you do buy protein supplements, here's what to look for.

Quality Protein

Dr. Peter Lemon of Kent State University in Kent, Ohio, rates Biological Value best for evaluating supplements: "The BV is based on the amount of a nutrient that is actually absorbed from the human intestine. So if you have a high BV protein that means that it has been measured in humans and a higher percentage of the nutrients are actually retained by the human as opposed to excreted. So it's really a direct measure of the value."

Here are the proteins to look for on the label, rated by their Biological Value, as published by the Food and Agricultural Organization of the United Nations:

Protein	Biological Value
Whey	952.9
Lactalbumin	942.8
Egg (whole)	943.2
Egg albumin	832.5
Casein	802.5
Soy	731.3

Carbohydrates

The same rules apply to protein powders as to sports drinks and bars. Fast-burning sugars are best immediately before, during, and after high-intensity workouts. They also help to get protein into muscles faster and better. I avoid high concentrations of fructose or corn syrup. The corn syrup is just cheap sugar while the fructose is more apt to make you fat than refill fuel stores. At other times of the day, mix protein powders with slow-burning carbos.

The following are some of the leading protein powders on the market.

Nitro Fuel Ion Exchange Whey Protein Powder
Twin Labs
Unflavored, unsweetened.

Pro:
- 100 calories.
- 25 grams of very highest quality ion-exchange whey protein.
- No fat, no filler, no sugars, no additives.
- Cleanest protein supplement out there.
- Allows you to add your own carbs.

MET-Rx Engineered Nutrition
MET-Rx
Available in Extreme Vanilla and Fudge Brownie.
According to MET-Rx, this product is in a category all its own: engineered food. It is formulated and assimilated for easy absorption by the body. The key ingredient, Metamyosyn™, is a unique protein blend that supplies the body with a powerful energy source for muscle regeneration and building.

Pro:
- 260 calories.
- 37 grams of protein.
- 2 grams of fat.
- 24 grams of carbohydrate.
- No sucrose or fructose added.

Con:
- 390 mg of sodium.

New Advanced Mass Fuel
Twin Labs
Available in Vanilla, Natural Chocolate, Strawberry, and Banana.

Pro:
- 50 grams of protein from high-quality milk and egg protein.
- Fat-free.

- Sugar-free.
- 100 grams of complex carbohydrate from maltodextrin.
- No simple sugars added.
- According to Twin Labs' Steve Blechman, New Advanced Mass Fuel taken after weight training "can speed recovery and produce a hormonal environment that, preliminary studies suggest, may be favorable to protein synthesis and muscle growth."

Con:
- 600 calories.

Shaklee Physique Workout Maximizer Supplement
Shaklee
According to Shaklee, this is really a recovery drink to be taken as soon as possible after exercise and, for serious athletes, also to be taken a couple of hours later. Available in Banana.

Pro:
- 320 calories.
- 21 grams of high-quality milk protein isolate and whey protein isolate.
- Less than 1 gram of fat.
- Over 99 percent lactose-free.
- Sugars are dextrose and maltodextrin.
- Full spectrum of vitamins and minerals.
- 37.5 micrograms of chromium.
- No fructose.

Parrillo Hi Protein Powder
Parrillo Performance
Available in Vanilla.

Pro:
- 105 calories.
- 20 grams of protein from calcium caseinate and soluble lactalbumin.
- Less than 1 gram of fat.
- 6 grams of fast-burning carbohydrate from maltodextrin.

- Fortified with 4 grams of free-form amino acids, including leucine, lycine, glycine, isoleucine, valine, cysteine, phenylalanine, methionine, and threonine.
- No fructose.

Joe Weider's Victory Pure Egg Protein
Weider Food Companies
Available in Natural Vanilla.

Pro:
- 140 calories.
- 20 grams of high-quality protein from egg albumin.
- No fat.
- 7 grams of fast-burning carbs from maltodextrin and glucose.
- Loaded with branched-chain amino acids (BCAAs) such as histidine, isoleucine, leucine, lysine, and many others.

Con:
- Contains fructose.

Hot Stuff Double X
Natural Health Products
Available in Banana and Chocolate. Because this product contains natural stimulants such as Siberian ginseng, guarana, and yerba maté, the company recommends ingesting it no later than 6 P.M.

Pro:
- 195 calories.
- 21 grams of high-quality protein from whey.
- Contains electrolytes.
- Contains branched-chain amino acids (BCAAs).
- Contains over fifty herbs.

Con:
- 15 grams of fructose.
- 5 grams of fat.

GETTING GREAT
FAST

Chapter 12

Old Warriors

IN THE LAST DECADE, ATHLETE AFTER ATHLETE IN SPORT AFTER SPORT HAS broken the mold. George Foreman won the heavyweight title at the age of forty-five. Nolan Ryan played major league baseball until age forty-six. Jimmy Connors made it to the semifinals of the U.S. Open at thirty-nine. Maurilio DeZolt won the Olympic silver medal for the grueling fifty-kilometer cross-country ski race at forty-one and the Olympic gold in the relay at forty-three. Francesco Moser set a world record for the mile on the bicycle at forty-two. While professional athletes have been disproving the conventional wisdom, the weekend warriors and fitness enthusiasts have missed out.

Conventional Wisdom:
> *If you're over thirty, give it up! You've had your day. Make way for the kids.*

New Paradigm:
> *Tilt the playing field to your maximum advantage — and win!*

Ask coaches and fans what they think about the over-thirty cyclist, skier, tennis, baseball, or football player. "Too old" is the likely response. Thirty-five and they've got one foot in the grave. But here's the truth. Sure, you may lose some ability with age, but it's less than you think. Thirty should be the halfway mark for an amateur athlete's career, not a dead end.

Older athletes are on the rise. Not only are they competing, the smart ones are winning. Even though the judges disagreed, Olympic fans knew that Torvill and Dean in their mid-thirties were simply the best ice dancers in the world.

HOW TO BEAT THE KIDS

When you compete against the kids, you're not on a level playing field. Synapses lose conductivity, making reflex time slower and movement less coordinated. University of California, Irvine, professor Dr. William McMaster points out that ligaments, tendons, and joint capsules stiffen, making you less fluid and supple. As a runner, your muscles will have stiffened, subtracting from your once-blistering pace. Your recovery time won't be as fast. This could pull a lesser man down. To tilt the playing field to your advantage, you need to leverage all your abilities with better equipment, technique, fueling, and training, as you'll find described in detail in the following chapters. Whether you couldn't care less about beating the kids or have Olympic aspirations, the same rules apply. Here they are.

Use Your Wallet

Better equipment, better training, better nutrition, better coaching, and better recovery cost money. All of them will make a big difference, and most of the kids can't afford them. You can't afford *not* to have them. Too expensive? The most expensive carbon fiber bike is a tiny fraction of the cost of angioplasty or bypass surgery. A new quiver of skis is cheaper than the increased premiums for health and life insurance of the severely sedentary.

Sidestep Your Weaknesses

Bill Clinton is a big guy. Running plays to none of his strengths. Jogging uses only a small fraction of his considerable muscle mass. His large frame is poorly designed to run much faster than an eight-minute mile. The age-related loss of springy, elastic muscle means a further drop in pace with time. Put Bill on rollerblades, a Stairmaster, or a mountain bike, and he'd be a killer. He could use much of his muscle mass, burn double or triple the calories, shed body fat, and radically improve his fitness. The natural elastic nature of a good stair machine, high-quality rollerblade wheels, or the frame, wheel rigging, and tires of a high-quality mountain bike more than compensate for nature's loss. An older athlete's biggest weakness will show up in sports where he fights the few unavoidable shortcomings of age or fights his basic anatomy.

Acquire Awesome Technique

By becoming a first-rate motor learner, you will pick up exquisite technique early and easily. This will catapult you past your younger rivals. Remember, kids "just do it." That translates to having no idea what they're doing, how they're doing it, or how to improve. Awesome technique optimizes how your body works to its best mechanical advantages with the least expenditure of energy.

Use Your Experience

Don't discount what you've learned in other sports. You're a treasure trove of knowledge that will let you outsmart the kids. If you are playing sports in your forties, you've played longer than many kids in their twenties have been alive. The pacing you've learned running translates to developing a sense of pace in mountain biking. If you've learned how to draft in cycling, you can apply that to a pace line of rollerbladers. If you've learned carbo loading and refueling techniques, you'll quickly translate that experience to new endurance sports. If your reaction time is off slightly in tennis, shorten your strokes to decrease your preparation time and use your experience to anticipate where the ball is coming. Older athletes anticipate far better than many younger ones.

Train Smarter

Do you ever wonder on the weekends why someone who puts in no more time than you blows past you? The answer is that he trains smarter. I'm as guilty as the next person of practicing the rat-on-the-treadmill mentality by rolling into the gym and doing the same workout day in day out, week in week out. That's training dumb, which leads to staleness, fatigue, and overtraining. Many older athletes attribute those symptoms to age instead of thoughtless training. Training smarter will increase your pace and endurance in compact training sessions. The most effective endurance training I've found is called anaerobic threshold training, aimed at increasing the speed at which you'll start making lots of lactic acid. I'll do twice-weekly forty-five- to sixty-minute race-pace sessions aimed at increasing that anaerobic threshold followed by two days of slower-paced recovery training. Over time, you'll be able to go faster and faster without the leg-burning, lung-searing effects of lactic acid.

Drink Rocket Fuel

Just when the kids start to fade away, you can power past them at a blistering pace if you have enough rocket fuel onboard. Kids may have the potential to be faster, but if they drop their blood sugar into the sewer, you've got 'em nailed.

Recover Faster

Recovery can sharply decline with age, while athletic function and skill are preserved. The good news is that recovery is one big area of your training that you can dramatically improve.

Sleep Like a Baby

Ever remember a good night's sleep as an early postadolescent? The accumulation of late nights, otherwise bizarre hours, alcohol, drugs, and a general sense of bewilderment robs many a youth of enough quality sleep to ever expect to do well. Great sleep takes serious planning, but the payoff is soaring productivity and terrific training. Poor-quality sleep cuts the intensity of your workouts by about 20 percent.

Build Stronger Muscles

Most kids don't weight train. You can beat the pants off them by having lots of explosive power and fresh young muscle.

Go for the Achilles

On one of the worst days of Vermont skiing in years, after rain and an ice storm in December 1993, I rode the chair with two post-adolescent young men. One said to the other, "Hey dude, how's your uncle Bud ski?" "Man, he does stuff I'd never do." "Yeah, but isn't he old?" "No man, Uncle Bud can ski me into the ground." After an extensive interview that lasted the length of the ski lift, I could understand the reasons why fifty-year-old Uncle Bud skied them into the ground.

Kids	Uncle Bud
Unfocused.	Focused.
Sports aren't important.	Sport is life.
No formal training program.	Disciplined training.
Lack of commitment.	Committed.
Lack of experience.	Massive experience.
Unaware of potential.	Fully exploited potential.
Empty wallet.	Full wallet.

Get In Early

Get into a new or obscure sport early, before the crowd does. Use your more advanced financial resources to get the cutting-edge technology and training to win. When the kids start clipping at your heels, get out! I did marathons in the mid-1970s, then triathlons, Iron Man contests, mountain bike racing, cross-country ski racing, speed-skate racing, Wintermeisters, and big-wave windsurfing each just a little ahead of the curve.

Play to Your Strengths

Given a choice, go for the sport that plays to all your natural strengths and abilities.

Buy the Best Toys

Skill-enhancement technology is the fastest way to become a legend. High-tech materials and computer-aided design leverage your skills and strengths to the maximum, teach you a higher level of play, and compensate for the weaknesses of age.

Play from a Quiver

At Sugar Cove in Maui, a group of men windsurf much as they play golf. Each has twelve or more different boards and ten different sails all rigged up and ready to go. Just like a golfer selecting exactly the right club for a shot out of a bunker, these guys call for their caddies to bring them their 7'6" left "asymmetrical" with a 4.5 slalom sail. If that's not quite right for the way the waves are breaking and the level of wind, the caddie does a quick swap from the quiver. That gives them a stunning advantage over the kids who just have one board. On Saturday mornings at Stowe, I'll put several pairs of skis by the lift. For a mogul run, I'll pull a mogul ski from the quiver. If I see someone rally fast in the lift line, I'll pull down a pair of super Gs. This allows the equipment to accommodate for whatever deficits age imposes.

Learn to Compensate

Tennis guru Vic Braden has found that as a person ages he loses literally just thousandths of a second in reaction time. Not much, but enough to make the difference between winning and losing. An older tennis player will lose thirty to forty-five milliseconds in reaction time in his small muscles. Good older athletes look exactly like young pros but with timing that's slightly off. How do they make up for it? Older men develop a system that doesn't need the split-second timing by cutting down a number of variables. Braden says, "Take, for example, a stroke in tennis. Rather than a young person like Agassi flying through the air using elbow and forearm rolls, an older man will leave his forearm still and swing from the shoulder, so he'll save time."

Protect Your Flank

Build up vulnerable body parts. Certain body parts are much more vulnerable to both overuse and underuse as you age. By hardening vulnerable body parts, you'll avoid most serious injuries.

Chapter 13

Sports-Improvement Technology

AS AN EXCHANGE STUDENT IN AUSTRIA DURING 1968, I RODE THE CHAIR-lift to the top of the Mutteralm ski area just outside Innsbruck late on a Saturday afternoon. With little grooming, lots of rocks, very firm ice, and immovable moguls, the skiing was really tough. Even the best skis of that period were as stiff as railroad ties and almost required a derrick to change direction. The man next to me on the lift was an engineer from Kneissl skis.

He pointed down at the huge number of awkward-looking skiers. Here, in the ski capital of Austria, almost everyone had his skis pointed downhill in a moderate snowplow or, at best, a stem christie. This was not the stuff of champions. He said, "Come back in ten years. All these people will make beautiful parallel turns. Not because they've gotten better, but because the ski will do it for them. Even couples in their seventies will ski like champions."

Twenty-five years have passed, and nearly everyone has his skis together in a nice parallel turn. Now, with little effort, most anyone can look pretty good on downhill skis. What this man looked into the future and saw was technology embedded in sports equipment that could increase the level of skill or play in sport. Now the technology of sports improvement has radically lowered the bar to excellence in tennis, skiing, cycling, golf, rollerblading, windsurfing, and a variety of other sports.

> Conventional Wisdom:
> *It's smart to be frugal when buying sports gear, especially if you're not good enough to take advantage of it.*
> New Paradigm:
> *Great technology creates great talent. Buy equipment for the athlete you'd love to become.*

Do you lust for the greatest new carbon fiber bike, the hottest new asymmetrical carving snowboard, the coolest new Andre Agassi tennis racquet? Buy it. Give yourself the permission to spend the money. Great equipment transfers the biomechanical advantages of the elite athlete to the amateur. You should have the best stuff, and this chapter will give you the perfect excuse to buy it!

It always rankles me when friends ask me what the cheapest bike or cheapest rollerblades or cheapest pair of tennis shoes is. More often than not, this individual really likes high-performance equipment. He drives an expensive car, plays a high-grade stereo, and wears hand-tailored suits, but he cheats himself at the sporting goods store. High-performance sports equipment makes a world of difference. A great bike makes you into a Ferrari. A seventeen-pound carbon fiber road bike will veritably jump when you stand up out of your seat. A cheap bike cheats you out of greatness. Many men buy bikes so heavy, unresponsive, and oppressive that they quickly retire them to the musty depths of their garage. Don't! An investment in a good piece of exercise equipment is a terrific investment in your health and your longevity. An investment in an expensive car, stereo, or meal won't make you live one day longer.

One big reason you may have performed poorly at sports as a kid is the equipment. Much of kids' athletic equipment is so poorly designed that it is nearly impossible to become proficient. My three-year-old son's bicycle weighed over fifteen pounds, only four pounds less than my adult racing bike! His tennis racquet is so stiff for his size and strength it's a wonder the racquet doesn't pull his arm off. If you have poor memories of trying to play tennis, ski, or roller-skate, just wait until you try the new technology. If your memories of trying sports as a kid are unfavorable, consider how much of your game will improve simply because today's technology is insanely great.

WHY YOU SHOULD BUY THE BEST

The best-designed sports equipment in the world works the way you do. Engineers take into account how muscles, joints, and ligaments actually work by examining limb speed and joint angles with computers. This equipment becomes a natural extension of the athlete. Top athletes demand this kind of equipment and they get it. Think of the elite athlete as the best judge of what really works. In each sports chapter I'll point out the key technology that will make you a better athlete. Here's a list of great reasons for buying the totally awesome new toys you've always wanted and what great technology can do for you.

Unleash Your Genius

Great technology lets you play up to the equipment. Take a good skier who doesn't really carve his turns. The radical new sidecuts on giant slalom skis allow him to roll easily onto a superbly carved ski. This skier might not otherwise ever learn to properly carve a ski despite lots of lessons and practice. All my life I've bought equipment that was much better than I was. I really believe that the equipment pulled me up, made me play up to its level.

Leverage Your Assets

Equipment is the ultimate equalizer. Another man may have more aerobic power or muscular strength, but equipment provides a lever that magnifies your own skills and transforms you into a first-class athlete. The key concept is the man-machine interface. Given your frame, strength, and level of ability, equipment offers you a powerful lever only if you are properly matched to it. I pay a lot of attention in this book to apparently small items: ski boot alignment in Alpine skiing, plate balance in rollerblading, frame flex in tennis. Perfecting the interface will give you a fast ride up the steepest learning curve. Ignore the technology and the interface to it and you'll be left behind. I had terrific ski-racing boots, the same ones that Alberto Tomba skis on. I also had the same skis he skis on, but my technique was badly flawed. Properly aligning my footbed and leg radically transformed me as a skier, making it incredibly easy to get on an edge and keep it.

Capture the Advantages and Genius of the Elite Athlete

Look at a great Alpine ski racer go through giant slalom gates. His skis carve at a 60-degree angle. He glides effortlessly from one extreme turn to another.

World-class skiers had to invent that technique. Once they did, equipment manufacturers had to design equipment to allow every racer to ski like that. Now you can buy that same equipment and capture the technical genius of the world's best. New boots that are very stiff side-to-side but quite flexible front-to-back let you move your legs and body from one turn to the next in a fraction of the time possible in recreational boots. Super-side-cut skis allow you to get up on a radical edge, just like the race photos show. Most men's gut reaction to "elite" equipment is that it's not for them, it's for the racer. To them I would say, capture the elite athlete's genius by using his technology.

Become a Fanatic

If you love great cameras, audio equipment, hunting, or fly-fishing gear, you've felt how equipment can draw you to an activity. Great sports gear provides tremendous motivation for fitness. There is no more perfect bonding of man and machine than equipment that extends his own abilities. That bond has an intoxicating quality that can drive you to a level of fanaticism about your sport.

Avoid Defeat

Inferior exercise equipment defeats many would-be athletes and fitness enthusiasts. Here's what I mean. As you exercise harder, equipment should ease the load on the body. Excellent equipment rewards you the faster you go. Poor equipment increases the workload way out of proportion to the modest increase in speed. Psychologically, you just won't put up with a lot more effort for a little more speed. That pegs your fitness level potential on the low side.

Many men feel they can't move faster than a crawl because they're on the wrong equipment. Here's an example. You bicycle on an old clunker. At naught point one miles an hour you're just fine. Your heart rate is probably a little above resting. You decide to really crank her up, but the workload quickly increases like a hill turning into a wall, with little increase in speed. Great equipment ensures that you can smoothly go up through the gears with the positive feedback of wind in your face, scenery whizzing by, and a gradually increasing demand on your heart rate and muscle, cruising up the power curve instead of crashing into it.

Keep Your Interest in the Game

Alpine skiing has had a unique run among sports. The tennis boom crashed. So did the racquet ball boom and the bicycling boom. The most interesting theory for this kind of crash is that the technology couldn't keep advancing the sport. The tennis boom died before the wide-body racquets. Had they been invented a few years earlier, men might have continued to advance to higher levels of play. Instead many were left frustrated intermediates and gave up the game. Since ski equipment has continued to advance, skiers have kept in the sport or come back to it. I left skiing for about fifteen years before a change in boot technology allowed me to overcome a fatal flaw in my technique. The new skis deliver amazing technical prowess from bottomless powder to steep icy hills. By getting the next generation of technology, you can improve your game substantially.

Overcome Limitations of Your Frame

If you feel you're too tall, too wide, too heavy, too short-legged, too knock-kneed, there's hope. Great sports and fitness equipment allows you to neutralize your deficits and magnify your assets.

WHAT TO LOOK FOR

Each individual sports chapter will give you the characteristics of the best sports equipment. This is a small sampling of what to look for.

Terrific "Feel"

This is the single most important ingredient in any piece of great sports equipment. Try a poor-quality stationary bicycle. At the 9 and 3 o'clock position, the workload is too easy. At the 12 and 6 o'clock position, the workload is too hard. The workload is hardest where it should be easiest. Your strength is trapped in poor bike design. Better exercise bikes accommodate for that weakness with heavy, high-tech flywheels.

Ergonometrics is the study of the human-machine interface. The best equipment makes certain that interface is nearly perfect. Equipment is very much like bionic limbs and joints. If it doesn't exactly mesh with your real joints and limbs, it'll feel terrible. Great technology is a perfect extension of your own body mechanics.

Decreased Workload

Automotive designers can just add a more powerful engine to make a car go faster. Humans need to make much more efficient use of their bodies to go faster, since they can't add lots of extra horsepower. That's accomplished in several ingenious ways.

Decreased Drag

The faster a runner, cyclist, skater, or skier goes, the more drag there is. The drag increases at a much faster rate than speed. That's why it takes so much more effort to go from 20 to 23 mph than from 2 to 5 mph on a bike. Some simple means of decreasing drag on a bicycle are to buy thinner tires and aerodynamic helmets. A more expensive way is an aerodynamic frame.

Lighter Weight

Graphite, boron, titanium, carbon fiber, and other materials bring great strength and resiliency with very low weight. That reduction in weight means that you can play harder with less strength. Lighter tips and tails make skis much easier to turn.

Decreased Inertia

Lighter bike rims are much easier to get going than heavier wheels. That one change in a bike lets you go much faster with the same amount of effort. Lighter ski tips and tails make turns easier to initiate because less effort is spent overcoming inertia. If you're going to pay for less weight, the most important weight to decrease is rotating weight, because it takes much more energy to get it moving and keep it moving. Heavy bike wheels, racquet heads, and ski tips all increase the effort it takes to move them out of proportion to their actual weight.

More Snap

Cheap equipment sucks away energy; great equipment gives it back. All the energy you throw into a cheap bike frame gets sucked up by the frame, making you increasingly tired. A high-tech carbon fiber frame will snap back after each downstroke, giving you more momentum. A dead ski will suck up all the energy you can put into it. A lively ski will throw that energy back into the next turn, improving your speed and the ease with which you ski.

Better Damping

Materials science allows the production of sports equipment that greatly reduces vibration. On a rough dirt road titanium bike frames soak up the shock. High-tech plastics curb the chatter felt in skis on ice and dampen the vibration felt on impact when striking a tennis ball. This allows you to play harder and longer and decreases your risk of injury.

Leveraging Power

Great sports equipment improves your leverage so that the same strength creates more power. The monocoque ski design delivers more edge-holding ability. A long, stiff rollerblading frame gives you much more push than the short, flexible plastic ones found on cheaper skates.

Leveraging Endurance

Heavy equipment requires so much power that you will quickly burn through energy stores and fatigue your high-end muscle fibers. Lightweight equipment lets your endurance muscle come into play, allowing you hours more activity.

Problem Solving

Many times equipment can solve a specific problem. I had a terrible time in mountain bike races across washboard sections. Despite bigger and bigger tires and front suspension, my aluminum frame made my teeth chatter. A titanium frame solved the problem. The shock absorption allowed me to buy smaller tires and lighter rims. Over a ten-mile race course, the bike improved my time by four minutes. In tennis, I simply could not get a long follow-through when hitting a hard ball using a stiff wide-body racquet. I changed to a very flexible, lightweight racquet, and now I can hit long through the ball, achieving depth and control. When looking to improve in sports, too many of us believe that it's all our fault. Often bad equipment gets in the way, while great equipment removes the roadblocks to greatness.

A FEW WORDS OF CONSUMER WISDOM

Look for Value

When you go from cheap equipment to good equipment, there is a drastic improvement in performance. By looking for the actual performance enhancements you can get very good value. The first performance increase in mountain bikes brings the weight down from thirty-two pounds to twenty-five. That twenty-five-pound bike is a very good value. Each pound after that has an enormous cost. For instance, to get a mountain bike from twenty-four pounds to twenty-one pounds can cost another $2,000. So look first for the improvements that give you the biggest performance boost.

Where to Buy

Looking for advice from a salesperson? Forget it! I'm so disappointed in American retail that I'm always amazed if someone will actually take the time to sell me an item. I look to specialty stores to buy equipment. A general sporting goods store often has few sales or service capabilities. A cartoon in one of the mountain biking magazines shows one bike store mechanic talking to another. He says: "You don't have to make it work, you just have to put it together."

I took my son to buy baseball gear at a large sporting goods chain store. We were introduced to a genuine "coach" who would help us out.

ME: Hi, I'd like to buy my son some baseball equipment.
SALESPERSON: It's over there.
ME: Well, what kind of a bat should I get?
SALESPERSON: One that's the right size.
ME: Well, how do I find the right size?
SALESPERSON: Try it out.
ME: Well, how do I try it out?
SALESPERSON (exasperated): Just try it out.

We bought him a bat, a glove, and a ball. The bat listed badly toward the ground. It was too heavy.

Fortunately, I went to another store, where a salesperson was quite helpful. The man explained to a baseball neophyte that my son should hold the bat out to the side with a straight arm at shoulder height to see if it was too heavy. Now that's not an awful lot of sports-specific knowledge to share with a customer, but get into high-tech bikes and skis and you are lost!

The Walk-Around

I bought some five-wheeled high-end rollerblades at a leading rollerblade shop in New York. Halfway around Central Park, one of the plates came undone. That could have resulted in a really bad fall. Another shop, which sells to national teams around the world, installed new screw holes on my skating boots. They were offset almost an inch too far to the inside. Boots that I bought from the top Australian company had the mounting screws offset one inch from each other, making it impossible to have the blades set symmetrically. New York City's premier bike-racing shop left a crank bolt undone. The crank came off halfway up a hill in Puerto Rico. This same shop fixed a derailleur problem but missed the fact that the rear chain stay was broken. When I sprinted up a hill, it mis-shifted, sending me onto the pavement. I lost two pints of blood. When you pick up new or repaired equipment, know what to check for. The bottom line is to make the most accomplished mechanic in town your best friend.

Beware of Mail Order

For simple items like skate wheels and bike helmets, a reputable mail-order company can be better than retail. But if it's anything that requires service, beware. I bought a fully suspended well-known make of premium mountain bike from a California bike shop as a test case to report on in this book. Everything that could go wrong did. The brakes rubbed on both sides, the spokes came up through the wheel wells to flat out the tires, the bottom bracket creaked and groaned, both crank arms loosened, it skipped in all the low gears, and the seat post broke. The brakes had so little stopping power that I crashed trying to stop on a flat bike path and suffered fifty stitches in the back of my head. The manufacturer tried and failed to make the bike right, then told me to take it to a local bike shop to get it in working order and then stiffed me for the $1,800 bill!

The lesson learned is simple: when you can't get face-to-face with the dealer or the manufacturer, you can write and call until you're blue in the face. What's the solution? Find the best mechanic you can. I did that at Toga, my local bike store. Find out what components he has had a good experience with, then ask him to build your bike and service it. If racers like Greg LeMond have learned one lesson, it's to find field-tested equipment that works under severe conditions and use that rather than ultratrick parts that are prone to fit poorly and break down.

Chapter 14

Rapid Skill Advancement

WITH DARK HAIRS BLEACHED BLOND BY LONG DAYS IN THE SUN, ASSISTED by several faint streaks of hydrogen peroxide, the physically perfect tennis instructor drills the ball over the net employing a natural flowing stroke. The ball lands precisely at your feet. You clumsily move out of its way, swing, and miss. The instructor smiles. His feigned graciousness is betrayed by a trace of smug self-satisfaction. Sure, his game is a joy to watch, but his subliminal message is clear: "I can do this and you can't." He's right, and that's the unfortunate message an overwhelming number of men take home from ski, tennis, golf, flying, fishing, and other lessons.

The instructor can play flawlessly and you can't. Why? He has absolutely no idea how he ever got as good as he did! "Gifted" or "natural" athletes learn as children by watching and imitating. They can't imagine why everyone can't learn the same easy way. They are clueless when it comes to how or why to teach someone in any other way than demonstrating their perfect form. Their "method," more often than not, is to demonstrate "doing it right" over and over without ever telling you how in a way you can understand. Picture-perfect instructors are the reason the majority of men don't like lessons, won't take lessons, and disdain instruction and instructors. They and their secondary school gym coach brethren are a big part of why 80 percent of American men don't do any meaningful physical activity. I never took a lesson at any sport until I was an adult. Instructors often intimidated me. I thought instructors were only for athletes who were already close to perfection and just needed some minor tuning up. The fact is that most adults don't learn best by watching, especially if humiliation is part of the game.

Conventional Wisdom:
You can't teach an old dog new tricks.
New Paradigm:
You can *teach an old dog lots of totally awesome great new tricks.*

Learning new skills is an invigorating, challenging, and rewarding intellectual activity. Acquiring a new set of skills fires more neurons, crosses more synapses, and takes more raw brainpower than the toughest calculus equation or advanced Latin translation. But, as contrasted to intellectual problem solving, learning new skills is tremendously satisfying and immediately rewarding. But the sad fact is that most adult Americans shy away from learning new skills because their whole upbringing rubs in the notion that it is just not possible unless you possess tremendous natural talent for sport. This is further borne out by endless failures in acquiring new skills. Yet brain scans of older patients with devastating strokes show enormous learning activity when they are taught new skills. Neurologists confirm that acquiring complex new skills is possible at any age. As a teenager, world champion tennis player Jim Courier was classified as someone who had difficulty acquiring skills. Many coaches wrote him off as an also-ran, not realizing that he had a style of learning strikingly different from most students.

Becoming a great learner is the cornerstone of good health and fitness. It will unlock a spectacular world of challenge, fun, excitement, and tremendous physical development. I have criss-crossed North America and Europe interviewing and being coached by the best teachers in the world. From that research, I am absolutely convinced that anyone can become a great learner. This chapter represents the best ways to do that. Learning to learn is the most exciting and interesting part of fitness today.

HOW TO GET GOOD FAST

Create an Image

To borrow a concept from Disney, if it can be imagined, it can be created. We build big mental walls against improvement because we can't imagine what we're trying to learn. Olympic-level ice skaters find they can't perform a triple axel jump until they can see it in their minds. Unless you have a mental image, regardless of how faint it is, you will not be able to perform the task at hand, because you will be blind to it. To use tennis as an example, start by observing the pros on TV and good players at your local club, or attend sporting events like the U.S. Open. I like watching real-life competition because it is in three dimensions, making it easier to see what's actually happening. Videotape at full speed is very difficult for the amateur to analyze. There are excellent videotapes that slow the motion down, pick it apart, and display the action at various angles. Look at still photos in books. Magazine editors go to great lengths to construct photomontages to show you where body parts are at each critical point. They're much easier to study and remember than a videotape. Read. Talk to good players and coaches off the court. Have them explain what they're doing and why they think it works.

When I go to sleep at night, I like to play back the images that I have created in various sports. Don't be concerned that the image you form is neither perfect nor as vivid as you might like. Think of it as a basic blueprint that will improve as you watch and play more of your new sport. It will give you a place to begin learning. Since so much of learning is error correction, it's all right if your mental image is wrong, because you can see and understand the error only if you have an image of it. By correcting it, your mental image grows in precision. You've improved your motor program. If you are a right-brained, visual learner, what I'm saying will make perfect sense because you think visually and can easily learn by watching. If you are a left-brained chunker, you may think I'm completely off the wall, but by opening your right brain's visual powers, you will create spectacular images as a basic frame around which to build your motor programs. One reason so many beginners at a sport look so lost is that they are operating in a vacuum. They don't have the analytical powers to really dissect what a coach is showing them, and they have no internal image as a frame of reference. Mental imagery provides detailed instructions on how to create mental images.

Don't be discouraged if you can't form images from visual references. Some people like myself are very poor at acquiring data that way. You may need verbal or written descriptions to paint a picture of the skill you wish to acquire. By the time you're finished, your visual image will have transformed itself from murky shadows to brilliant Technicolor.

Get on Your Marks

When a sprinter takes his mark, it's not part of some bizarre ritual. This is the best position from which to accelerate. That's what those "marks" are for; they prepare the body for action.

When you first try to execute a new movement, you have a huge range of possible motions to make, like a person flailing his arms as he first jumps out of an airplane. Achieving a good starting position limits those movements by getting each limb in the best position from which to spring into action. Look at top professional golfers, skiers, and tennis players when they are in their "ready stance." They look almost statuesque in their perfection. A good "ready stance" is a terrific shortcut. You can practice it in the mirror at home and make corrections until you have a perfect ready position, bringing you a long way toward building a good motor program.

For each sport, I'll list very specific, easy-to-remember marks. For instance, in Nordic skiing it's "toes-knee-nose" before the beginning of each stride. That means that you could drop a weighted line from your nose through your knee to your toes. When I start skiing at the beginning of every season, I'll look down the end of my nose to make certain that it's aligned over my knee and toes before beginning the next stride. That easily sets up the correct alignment to prevent making a mistake before beginning a stride.

Try getting "on your marks" so that you can do it without thinking about it. Since the limbs and muscles are not in motion, you have lots of time to make certain that every body part is exactly where it should be. Just think about striking the perfect pose. Close your eyes and develop a mental picture of where every body part is based on where you feel it is. I was really struck watching John McEnroe in person at the U.S. Open. He looked almost robotic in the precision with which he moved and positioned himself before each service. You could tell that he had clearly constructed an exact image of what his starting position should be. Great coaches will tell you that many poor shots are generated by a poor starting position.

Learn Cues to Guide You

Once you are on your marks, each body part has a specific path through which it should travel to properly execute a skill. I like very specific cues I can think about as I perform. For a tennis forehand, I may think about reaching my palm out through the ball and then up over my left shoulder after my arm is extended. These cues should be simple enough to execute. Most people can handle only one or two cues at a time. You'll know how good the cues are by how well they work.

You can pick cues up from tips in magazines or from good players and coaches. No cue is perfect. A good cue simply gets you closer to a correct motion. Further correction by a good coach will let you perfect an exacting groove for your new skills. Even with no mental image of what you're doing, good cues will get you started in the right direction. Even Olympians continue to use them to keep their performance at its best. As you get better, you can use sequenced cues that take you step-by-step throughout an entire motion.

Get Good Error Correction

The very best way to learn is to get regular feedback from a coach who will tell you accurately about very specific errors and then pat you on the back when you correct each one. Complex feedback is totally useless and incomprehensible to most students. That doesn't mean you're stupid. It means your instructor doesn't know how to teach you. It's easy to single out those coaches. They're testy and irritable when you're just "not getting it." Of course, you don't understand what he wants because you don't know what he's saying! Corrections should be simple. You should be able to think about the correction during your next attempt. For example, you might be asked to keep your elbow close to your body or keep your head steady so that it doesn't "jerk up" on impact when you hit a tennis ball. Those are cues you can actually think about while you're performing a skill. As each one of these corrections sticks, it becomes incorporated into your motor program. These corrections may be visual, where your instructor will show you your error and then show you the right way. Or your instructor may tell you to try for a certain "feel." Cues help most where the instructor tells you to move a hand, elbow, shoulder, hip, or other body part in a specific way. You try to follow the cue, and the instructor then imitates your error, demonstrates the correct technique, and then gives you cues to perform the skill the correct way yourself.

Error correction is just like sculpting. With each subtle change, you get better and better. You'll become eager for error correction, knowing it's the best way to learn rather than a mark of humiliation. Make certain you fully understand the correction. If you don't know what you've done, there is no learning. It's only with a "knowledge of your performance" that you will improve. That's why lots of men think they can never get better. They don't want the constant criticism of a wife or friend or coach who points out their errors, so they don't listen. They don't want to be "bugged," don't like instructors, and so never improve. Learning takes place quickly and will really stick if you get good error correction. It is the very essence of learning. I view a good motor-learning experience as better than psychotherapy. A psychotherapist might convince you that you're okay when you're really a mess. After a coaching session, you really are better than you were before! How many psychiatrists can claim that kind of success after an hour of psychotherapy?

Good students of motor learning don't just like feedback, they love it. They'll be motivated to try harder. So much so that it's sometimes pretty hard to get away from a coach and play on your own. That's why I think it's critical to develop the next step, your own internal sense of reward for what you do.

Trial and error really is the best way to learn. Get an idea of what you want to do. Do it. Then learn from errors you've made. Those errors won't be hard to see. Even professional athletes make large, easy-to-see errors. Curiously, those who make big errors and have them corrected may have much better long-term learning than those who perform a skill right off the bat, because they are more likely to forget it and be unable to perform it in the future. So if you've tried long and hard to water-start a windsurfer in big seas, when you've finally got it, you've got it forever. Twenty years from now, you could head back out and do it again. Correcting big errors is the best way to set skills in stone. Without error correction, you'll learn nothing.

If you think you're setting yourself up for getting criticized, that's not what error correction is about. Good error correction motivates students to practice longer, harder, and better. It also reinforces what you've done right.

Go to the Videotape

Some of your best error correction will come from your own analysis. I took my 8 mm video camera to tape my tennis game last December. I was just astounded at what I saw. On my backhand, I leaned down with my upper body and then used my upper body to scoop up the ball. Ouch! Even though I thought I had corrected my forehand backswing so that it went back 55 degrees, on the videotape it was 200 degrees. No wonder I had no time to get prepared! Now these are two huge errors that I should have overcome long ago. I know what I want to look like now that I have a solid mental image of what I did wrong and how to correct it. Curiously, even those who claim to have poor mental-imagery skills can see how far off their form is from what they think it should be. Videotape is a great motivator. New cameras with LCD screens on the back let you review your performance on the court or slope. Even in the viewfinder you'll get a good picture of what you're doing wrong. Use the pause button to compare what you see to still photos of great athletes. You'll be surprised at how quickly your own analytical skills will build.

Tune in to Onboard Feedback

The human body is wired with the most elaborate internal feedback systems of any device on the planet. Each muscle and joint feeds your brain up-to-the-millisecond information on where each limb is and what it's doing. The human brain can gather millions of pieces of data about joint position, muscle force, and limb velocity with astonishing speed and accuracy and analyze it instantaneously. The trouble is, most of us were never trained to pay any attention to this data. In fact we're likely to mistake totally where our limbs are and what they're doing! Nearly every pro athlete questioned will say he performed a skill in a specific way when the cameras showed the opposite! Learning how to use your onboard sensors means that you can learn to correct your own errors, a tremendously powerful learning tool.

Here's how. After executing a skill, say a tennis backhand, spend about five seconds tuning in to your onboard position sensors. What position were your limbs in? At what angles were your joints? Where do you think you went wrong? Your eyes can tell you where a ball went. Your ears can tell you if it was mishit on the racquet. Your muscles can tell you how much power you applied. Once you've got the picture, ask your coach for verification. When you get your internal feedback to reflect accurately what the coach or video camera sees, you'll have acquired the greatest learning skill of all. Then you will become your own best coach. Here are the senses you should concentrate on:

Visual. Your eyes give you a three-dimensional picture of your entire playing field. You get feedback on what you have accomplished. You made it around the slalom gate; you hit the tennis ball deep into the crosscourt by the baseline. Visual feedback lets you know if you achieved what you hoped to. You can also see certain motions, such as arm and hand position at the end of a tennis forehand.

Power sense. You have millions of tiny receptors in muscles to tell you how tense they are and how much power you are applying. You can learn to get the right "feel" for the correct amount of power required to perform skills.

Position sense. Tendons and ligaments have position receptors that tell your brain exactly where they are. Most of us are blind to these position receptors. However, if you develop "onboard feedback," you'll sense the error you made before your coach tells you what it was. In fact, you should take a moment at the end of a golf stroke, tennis shot, or ski turn to assess what you think you did, before your coach tells you what you actually did. This helps you sharpen your position sense. A great way to start learning position sense is to "get on your marks" with your eyes closed. Use your position sense to put your arms, legs, and trunk in their proper position. Now look at yourself in the mirror. The closer you can merge your visual system with your onboard sensors, the better position sense you will develop.

Play It Back

After you finish practice, take the mental image of the skill you're acquiring and refine it with the new experiences you've just had. Use any new cues that you've learned as you replay the action in your brain. Try to feel where your limbs are as you execute a skill. Assemble all your new data and create a new, improved image. Don't be concerned that it's hard to see at first. Your mental-imagery powers will rapidly improve as you learn to visualize better. This is the best way of tying together what you've learned into a newer, better motor program that will really stick.

If you're skeptical about the power of imagery, science can prove you wrong. Students who practiced a sports skill through mental imagery were able to perform that skill just as well as those who practiced the real skill!

Make a Checklist

Even Olympic champions use checklists. Tommy Moe, during his Olympic gold medal downhill ski run at Lillehammer in 1994, had a two-point checklist: hands out in front, pressure on the downhill ski. He credits using just those two points with his victory. Figure skater Brian Boitano attributes his fall during the same Olympics to a failure to use his technical checklist.

I make notes after a lesson, a workout, or reading an article or viewing a videotape. I use these notes to make a checklist for my next practice session. I'll choose several items and then scan myself during play to make certain that I'm doing them. For instance, in Alpine skiing, I'll scan to make certain my shoulders are level, that my hands stay relaxed and low in front of me, that I go forward onto the balls of my feet in the beginning of the turn, then to my arch in the center, and finally to my heel at the end. The scan will concentrate on just one item for several turns. Once it checks out, I'll move to the next. This method refines each item until it's finally fully automatic.

Learn How You Learn

The steps above represent several different ways of learning. Some may make perfect sense to you. Others may seem strange or undoable. That's because each one of us has learning methods that we like best. My brother-in-law Brad Allinson can watch a tennis match on TV and then replicate the play on the court. Others simply need to be left alone to experiment and feel how to perform a new skill.

So why present so many different ways of learning? Although you'll learn best in one way, you'll become a far better motor learner if you tune in to other methods to refine your skills. They won't help you as much at the start as your own natural style, but they will help you perfect your skills.

Remove Physical Impediments

Make sure you build the power, speed, and balance to acquire the movement patterns you'll need. At the beginning of any sport, you probably won't be hampered by lack of physical strengths and skills, but you will be as you get better. Make certain that you remove these choke points before they become a problem. For instance, in rollerblading, skiing, and tennis, you'll need to be able to lower your thighs until they are parallel to the ground and still be strong enough to explode from that position on one leg. That's the basis of power in all three sports. You may choose to work on a Stairmaster and do leg presses to build that strength.

Think Biomechanics

There is a great misconception that form in sport is what counts. That's just hogwash. The way you move your body or limbs should be based on the most effective way to use your muscles. This is the science of biomechanics. You should in every sport think about why what you are doing makes sense. For instance, tennis players are asked to get in the ready position by raising their elbow. It feels odd and looks weird until you realize that you are simply lifting your upper arm to the top of a pendulumlike arc, adding energy to the shot as the racquet falls. A prominent skiing magazine put an instructor on the front cover with a great big I-can-do-this-and-you-can't grin. His form looked perfect, with his body facing directly downhill, his hand held out from his body, his poling hand cocked out. However, if you looked at the bottom of the picture, you could see he was skidding his skis. Great form, but terrible function. Don't let coaches stamp you out of a cookie cutter! Your anatomy and physiology allow you to do best in a highly individual way. Find it!

FINDING THE RIGHT COACH

Learning doesn't have to take very long at all if you can really connect with your coach or instructor. From the first minutes of a lesson, you should be able to implement each suggestion the coach makes and then refine it through error correction.

Teaching Style

Master tennis coach Vic Braden likes to talk about people who learn by seeing, doing, feeling, or thinking. One of these will be your strong suit. Choose a coach who can give you information in the way you understand best. If you are a visual learner, then a coach can simply demonstrate. If you're not a visual learner, then you'll be blind to the instructor's "follow me" charge down the ski slope, since you won't be able to follow complex movement patterns and discern much usable information.

You need a coach who can watch you and offer simple corrections for what you are doing wrong. Too often a frustrated instructor shouts a continuing volley of commands about what you should do rather than correcting what you shouldn't do. That's why you should aggressively seize the driver's seat when you take a lesson of any kind. Don't stand there like a sheep going to slaughter. Be a good consumer. Tell the instructor how you learn best.

Attitude

Coaches can be really prickly. One coach, in his mildly insulting manner, commented on how much better my backhand was than my forehand. I answered him, "Yeah, it's more expensive." I explained that I've spent a lot more money on my backhand than my forehand. He didn't see the humor. Instructors who are heavily critical and too caught up in their own glory are generally useless. Coaches first need to motivate. That means conveying a really positive attitude.

Results

An instructor shouldn't be judged on how well he plays but on how well he gets you to play. Judge a teacher by his product. I've never seen the famous tennis coach Nick Bollettieri play a game, but he has produced Jim Courier, Andre Agassi, and a swarm of hot new prospects. He and his staff endlessly and selflessly think about the game, think about why the pros hit the ball a certain way, and think about how to get off-the-street students to follow suit.

Cues That Make Sense in a Language You Can Understand

The best single article I've ever read in a tennis magazine was by Nick Bollettieri in *Tennis Match* about the elbow in ground strokes. This article made a simple point about where the elbow is in relation to the rest of the body. You lead back with your elbow first like Ivan Lendl, and you keep your elbow close to your side. It was information you could take right out to the court to improve your forehand because the cues were so simple. When you're looking for an instructor, look for someone that can give you good clear cues.

TRY A NEW SPORT

Most men are set in their ways when it comes to sports skills. They have a hard time accepting criticism or coaching because their motor programs for those sports are set in stone. By trying new sports you're forced to develop new frames of reference. Rollerblading, windsurfing, and snowboarding all teach you how to learn. You'll develop onboard error correcting that allows you to improve vastly in sports you've done longer.

Windsurfing is the ultimate motor-learning sport. It's really not exactly like skiing, surfing, sailing, rollerblading, or any other sport you've ever tried. Sure, you'll be able to use bits and pieces of all those sports. Skiing helps with the knee position in jibed turns. Surfing helps with carving down the face of a house-high wave. Rollerblading helps with shifting your hips. Sailing helps with a feeling for the wind and sail. But you will be surprised that nothing comes automatically in windsurfing. I've never seen someone just jump on a board and do it. You've got to create brand-new motor programs. That's what's so frustrating and yet so helpful about windsurfing. I've never yelled louder or cursed more foully than when learning to windsurf. I encourage anyone to try windsurfing because it gives you such a fine appreciation for how to learn sports. You'll be much more receptive to learning tennis, golf, or whatever else you want to try.

Chapter 15

Training Smart

ALBERTO TOMBA, THE MOST FAMOUS SKI RACER IN THE WORLD, BRAGS that he sleeps until noon, trains at the beach, and parties with five women until 3 A.M. on race day. Some years Alberto wins, others he's lucky if he finishes. Why the inconsistency? Training dumb. Athletes in their twenties think they can get away with poor training habits. Sometimes they do, but most never trained as smart as they could. Older athletes can't afford to train dumb, but they have tremendous wisdom and experience they can carry from sport to sport. What is it that men want to know most about training? At cross training clinics in Vail, Colorado, the most frequently asked questions by forty-five-year-old men are the following:

- How do I train more efficiently with my time?
- How can I get much better without giving up my day job?

The answer is simple: train smarter than the kids.

> Conventional Wisdom:
> *No pain, no gain.*
> New Paradigm:
> *No brain, no gain.*

WHY YOU SHOULD TRAIN SMART

Training isn't a black hole into which you deposit time and hope for a reasonable outcome. Science knows precisely what you'll get out of every hour you train.

You'll Recover Faster

Serious triathletes often train so long and so hard that they're fried by race time. Those who plan for recovery come out of the blocks to beat those with superheavy training schedules.

You'll Avoid Injury

Ninety percent of overuse injuries are due to poor training. Men who complain about shinsplints have often failed to follow the most rudimentary training plan.

You'll Gain Speed

Men who train part-time often maintain the same workout intensity year in and year out. By adding one or two days a week of "threshold" training, they can substantially increase their pace without the risk of injury.

You'll Increase Endurance

Strategically planned training allows you to increase endurance without big increases in time spent training.

You'll Become Efficient

Elite-class triathletes bike five hundred miles, run one hundred miles, swim twenty miles, and put in four hours in the weight room each week. But who has that kind of time? Smart triathletes are staying very competitive with a fraction of this amount of training time by getting maximum effect for the training they do.

You'll Stay Young

Overtraining makes you age. Training smart keeps you young.

WHAT REALLY WORKS

Training smart means that you aim for and get a very specific effect. Training dumb is training without a plan and without a goal.

Cross Training

Training in at least one alternate sport allows you to sharply reduce the amount of overuse while maintaining a very high level of conditioning. Cross training has gained in popularity because more men want diversity in their training. Frank Shorter has had his longest injury-free training period by cross training. He does his intensity training in his sport of running, but he then does his long slow distance on a bicycle, thereby taking away 2.5 hours of pounding each week. One of the best ways to use cross training is to avoid the pointless hammering of longer, slower distances so you have the energy and injury-free fitness to really hammer during hard training days. Even Greg LeMond will give up his bike to cross-country ski or rollerblade.

Varied Training

There is no more telling trait of the over-thirty athlete or fitness enthusiast than the desire to undertake the same workout every day: the same distance, the same pace, the same sport. Part of this is out of a fear of deconditioning or gaining weight. But the real problem with the sameness is that it leads to overtraining, staleness, and boredom. Many men are uncertain how to vary a program and lack the time to figure it out. A very modest amount of planning pays off in big gains without injury or overtraining. The most important planning is within a given week where each high-intensity training session is followed by two easier ones.

Heart-Rate Monitors

You wouldn't drive a sports car without a tachometer, and you shouldn't train without a heart-rate monitor. This is the smartest way to train. You'll know exactly what you've done and can measure the results.

Increasing Your Anaerobic Threshold

There has been only one really revolutionary training concept in the last twenty years: anaerobic threshold (AT) training. By moving your

AT you can go faster in any endurance activity. Moving the AT should be the first and major speed goal of any endurance training program. Thirty to forty-five minutes of near-race-pace training once or twice a week is the most commonly used routine.

Hard/Easy/Easy Training Days

Training works only if your body has a chance to adapt to it. A hard day followed by two easy days is the surest way to get as fast as you can and recover the best you can.

Biomechanical Efficiency

Great technique delivers a huge energy savings. By concentrating on learning great technique you can sharply increase your speed without an increase in training. For instance, in Nordic skate skiing, you can double your speed by employing a mechanically correct position. Getting your hips to move forward alone creates huge energy savings and big increases in speed.

GENERAL GUIDELINES

Start Slowly

The East Germans had the most successful Olympic teams in the world. Their great secret was knowing how to train athletes. Their most telling principle was that of slowly building a large base before undertaking high-intensity training. Too many people who take up fitness are pushed too hard too fast. The truth is, if you're in it for the long haul, it doesn't matter how slow a start you get. The harder you start, the harder you'll fall. Too much early intensity promotes injuries and dropout. I took years to build up any kind of volume, beginning with one-mile walks with my father.

Warm-ups

Warm-ups and stretching are often confused. I've exercised for decades without stretching. I've come to view pre-exercise stretching as a near-religious ritual. For runners, it appears to be an obsessive-compulsive disorder. In truth, I think stretches make a poor warm-up. Studies have shown that they create more injuries than they prevent when muscles are cold and stiff. A muscle shouldn't be stretched until it's warm and pliable.

But what about the warm-up? Is there a rationale? In fact, there are two. First, muscles don't deliver as much energy unless they are run at a higher-than-resting-state temperature. You just won't go as fast if you start out your training session full throttle with cold muscles, and you may tear a muscle. Muscles perform poorly until they reach the proper temperature, just as car engines do. Second, if you start without a warm-up, you may cause an irregular heart rhythm, especially if you exercise in the morning. Even a seventeen-year-old will have heart-rhythm irregularities without a good warm-up. The best warm-up is just beginning your workout slowly.

I like to take the first five to ten minutes of exercise at a leisurely pace, say 50 percent of maximum heart rate. It should feel easy, comfortable, and unforced. If you find a muscle group is too stiff to go all out, then is the time to stretch it. For speed skating, I do four miles at a moderate pace, then really stretch my back. A stretched muscle feels terrific after a warm-up whereas it can feel brittle before. After ten minutes I gradually pick up the pace. When I check my heart-rate monitor recording after such a workout, I find much higher sustained heart rates with a good warm-up.

WHEN TO EXERCISE

Early

Early in the morning, exercise is certainly possible, but your body is at such a physical low point that you may feel you're working twice as hard to go the same speed as during an afternoon workout. Here's why. Your adrenaline, blood pressure, and many of your body systems are at a low ebb. Any activity can be a big jolt to the body. Most heart attacks and strokes occur in the mornings. The only advantage of exercising in the morning is that it gives you an extra spike in your peak daily energy level. This gives you an artificial midmorning peak from your morning workout and a real one in the early afternoon from your body clock. If you have no other choice, you're better off exercising in the morning than not at all. It's also the best way to schedule exercise so that you have the fewest social, family, and work conflicts.

At Noon

A number of major corporations — Exxon, Bonnie Bell, and Johnson & Johnson are a few — encourage their employees to exercise at lunchtime because they know it will improve their afternoon productivity and general health. They make it all the easier by providing exercise facilities and programs. Johnson & Johnson, for example, has erected a large bubble-covered exercise facility for its employees in New Brunswick, New Jersey. Workers there can take advantage of supervised exercise classes and workouts on strength-training equipment and a small indoor track, as well as of instruction in nutrition and the control of cigarette, drug, and alcohol abuse. Some companies even pay their employees to exercise at lunch. If you exercise just before lunch, your adrenaline level will remain high, so you won't be as hungry — a big plus for weight-watchers. New evidence from Cornell University indicates that if you exercise within a couple of hours after eating, you may burn off more calories than if you exercise on an empty stomach. So either way, you win.

In the Afternoon

This often coincides with the body's natural peak for your best workout time. It also gives you an energy boost that lasts through the evening and will kill some of your appetite for dinner.

In the Evening

If you exercise less than four hours before you go to bed, you may have trouble falling asleep, since exercise causes your body temperature to rise for up to six hours. Sleeping calls for a lowered body temperature. If you time your workout exactly, your body temperature will be dropping nicely at about the same time you want to go to sleep, making your exercise a natural sleeping pill. Regular exercise also improves the quality of your sleep. The more you exercise, the more deeply you'll sleep, and it's deep sleep that makes you feel the most refreshed and keeps you young.

HOW MUCH TO EXERCISE

The American College of Sports Medicine says that you need twenty to sixty minutes, three times a week, at 60 percent of your maximum capacity, and they're right. That, however, is not as difficult as it seems. If you do the sport you love for an hour each day on the weekends, you're more than halfway there. You need not do all your exercise at one time during the day. I divide mine up by cycling or skating to work in the morning, then taking a longer circuit home at night. Twenty minutes at either end of the day is pretty easy to get your mind around.

If you exercise less than three times a week, you may not get an adequate aerobic benefit. If you exercise more than five times a week, you will receive only very small additional increases in physical fitness and there's a much greater chance of injury. Spacing workouts throughout the week — every other day — may give you the best results with the least risk. I've always worked out seven days a week but divided up my training into different sports.

If you really get into an aerobic sport, you'll base your exercise on the distance you cover each week. For instance, a marathoner might run sixty miles a week, a cyclist might bike two hundred miles a week, a swimmer might log nine miles a week. Pure volume of exercise is what builds up your heart, lungs, ligaments, tendons, and muscles to withstand high-intensity exercise. It's very important when you begin a sport just to build distance and not worry about intensity. That's especially true for high-stress activities like running. You need to be careful to build your volume by about 15 to 20 percent per year so you don't suffer overuse injuries. For pure fitness, there's no need ever to do very intense training.

MEASURING THE EFFECTS OF EXERCISE

I'm a big believer in heart-rate monitors. They're pretty inexpensive now and a great way to measure intensity. I find myself really coasting without one; I won't work my heart much more than 110 beats a minute. But using a heart-rate monitor like a race car driver does a speedometer, I'll push myself to 160 beats per minute on a hard day, 170 in competition. Much has been made of staying within a target zone whose boundaries are defined by your age, but there's a fairly wide heart-rate variation at any given age. You'll also find your heart rate will vary tremendously from sport to sport, so you'll want to figure a good range for each one. The top end of that predicted heart rate is a pretty reliable red line that indicates you've overdone it. Most of us never get up there. The heart-rate monitor keeps you honest. It's a great way to evaluate a new activity. The monitor's cost is now below $100. I use a Polar Vantage because I can download the results into my computer. I wear it as a wristwatch, then put the chest band on for exercise. Here's the table that shows the general range for heart rate.

Age:	20	30	40	50	60	70	80	90	100
100%	200	190	180	170	160	150	140	130	120
90%	180	171	162	153	144	135	126	117	108
80%	160	152	144	136	128	120	112	104	96
70%	140	133	126	119	112	105	98	91	84
60%	120	114	108	102	96	90	84	78	72
50%	100	95	90	85	80	75	70	65	60
40%	80	76	72	68	64	60	56	52	48

- 100% is pretty hard to hit and impossible to maintain.
- 90% is what really top athletes can maintain on race day.
- 80% is what you'll want to hit on your one or two hard days a week, once you're in really good condition.
- 70% is the practical top end for general fitness.
- 60% is what you need to hit for a good workout.
- Below 50% and you're coasting. A recent *New England Journal of Medicine* study shows that only vigorous activity provides a big leap in protection against heart disease.

Get a sense of what your heart rate is at specific speeds in your sport. I like knowing that because it tells me when I've still got enough oomph to pick up the pace or warn me if I'm at red line. For instance, 22 mph is a pretty good solo clip on a road bike; 26 mph is what you'd expect in a pack; 30 mph is the world record for an hour; 34 mph is what Greg LeMond and others average during the Tour de France. One last reason for a heart-rate monitor. It really allows you to compete with yourself. When the monitor ticks the top of the scale, you know you're doing your best. Even if you get passed, you will know you're as good as the competition in terms of your own personal effort.

In our sports science laboratory at the 1980 Winter Olympics in Lake Placid, we measured the top speed at which athletes could go without crashing. We called this the anaerobic threshold (AT), because faster speeds would drive major muscle groups to make enormous amounts of harmful lactic acid. Exercise right at that threshold twice a week for thirty to forty-five minutes is the single most reliable means of improving the overall tempo of your workouts and the speed at which you can compete or rip off body fat. Although there is no good self-administered test, you can get a good sense of where your anaerobic threshold is by determining your race pace for a thirty- to forty-minute event such as a ten-kilometer road race or a fifteen-mile bicycle time trial. You'll find that the threshold occurs around the point where you have a nice heavily winded sensation but short of air hunger. It's just past the point where you can carry on any kind of conversation. Once you pass over the threshold, you'll quickly build up too much lactic acid and be forced to slow or stop. To be frank, only sophisticated lactic acid or computerized gas analyzers in sports science labs can precisely locate the AT, but you can approximate this point by increasing the intensity of your exercise every couple of minutes until you get to that nice evenly winded state. Be sure to use a heart-rate monitor. I found, for example, that I can race a bike at a heart rate of 167 for forty-five minutes. That's a good approximation of my AT. By the time I hit 175, I know I'm good only for several minutes. You'll quickly get a sense of the highest continuous heart rate you can maintain for each activity. Cyclists can get a very approximate AT by having a local coach administer the Marconi test, which relies on measuring heart rates continuously as you increase your workload.

Why is the AT so critical? Dr. William Kraemer, director of research at the Center for Sports Medicine at Pennsylvania State University, answers: "The value of knowing about anaerobic threshold is that as athletes get in better and better shape they can go harder and harder without running into excessive production of lactic acid. Your VO_2 MAX doesn't have to change at all. But if you push from 55 to 75 percent or 75 to 85 percent, where you start really producing a lot of lactic acid, you're getting really fit. The Olympic Committee presented a paper showing that they found no increase in VO_2 MAX but performance was improved with the key being anaerobic threshold which was pushed much higher. As these competitive cyclists aged, their VO_2 MAX decreased, but their anaerobic threshold went up and their proficiency went up. So they were performing better because of the AT, not the VO_2 MAX." Bottom line: older athletes can get better and better only by improving their AT, not their VO_2 MAX, which is fixed in early adulthood. Untrained men have ATs of around 50 percent. Trained athletes range from 75 percent to over 90 percent of VO_2 MAX. When a great runner is at a five-minute mile, he may not be exerting anywhere near the effort of an eight-minute-mile runner. Why? The faster runner is still running comfortably below the level where he makes painful levels of lactic acid, while the slower, less fit runner has shot right past his AT and his lungs and legs are burning. But as the slower runner improves with training, he'll feel less and less effort at higher and higher speeds because his AT has increased. A high anaerobic threshold allows you to use all you've got.

For the last several years the popular press has written a great deal about low-intensity workouts. The conventional wisdom is that they are better for you because they burn more fat, they're safer, and you get just as much of a cardiovascular workout. Now here's the truth. Sure, you'll burn more fat than carbohydrates at a very low intensity.

So if you're walking and burning 200 calories an hour, over half will be fat, or roughly 100 calories. But if you were exercising at 1,600 calories an hour, you might burn 700 calories of fat. The only way to get to a 1,600-calorie workout is with high-intensity race-pace training once or twice a week. Still, the rest of your training should be at a much lower intensity, so you can recover. The Australian cycling team spends 90 percent of its time below 120 beats a minute. That's practically a standstill compared to American cyclists. If you train one or two really easy days for every hard one, the hard one will be much faster and far more effective than if you hit the wall every day. That's because you recover so much more effectively. New research by Dr. Dave Costill at Ball State University appears to show that older athletes will actually lose the muscle fibers that make them fast if they don't use them. Men who only train slow will become permanently slow.

Exercise has gotten a bad reputation because it appears painful to even the most casual observer. Ever watched Olympians at practice on a speed-skating oval or sliding across a cross-country ski course? Do they look pained or hurt? No way! The better you get, the less exertion you perceive at any given level of exercise. When you begin, every motion seems painful. There's a reason you feel pain: your body is telling you to take it easy. Let your body accommodate to the strain you're putting on it. If you're not shooting for the Olympics, there's never a need to suffer serious discomfort when you exercise. Just pay attention to your perceived exertion. Rate your workouts. Back off when it hurts. Give yourself several days of slow workouts. When you go hard, it should be because your muscles feel restless, itching — even anxious — to get a great workout.

DRESSING THE PART

In dressing for your sport, you have two options. You can really get into the look with the latest, hottest fashions. This helps lots of people "psyche themselves." Some of it's also pretty functional. But there is another school of thought. Recently, the government performed a survey and discovered that people who didn't exercise were intimidated by the Lycra look. Those individuals may want to dress down.

The best way to dress down is to find the most comfortable clothing. I'm a big believer in cross-sport dressing. I wear my bicycling gear for speed skating, my surfing shorts for cycling, soccer gear for mountain biking. That allows you to be comfortable, look serious, and still display a certain disdain for those that are "too serious" or too self-important about their sport.

Many people give up exercising during the winter. That's a big mistake. Just when gloom and doom set in, just when you're most tempted by the holidays to overeat, you give up exercise. The Scandinavians have the best slogan: "There's no such thing as cold weather, just cold clothing." You can dress for any weather. I commute by bicycle all winter. That's made possible by a terrific winter jacket and pants with a Gore-tex front but a back that breathes so I don't overheat. I'm a big believer in layering the new synthetics to keep dry and warm. Capilene, Polypro, and Supplex are a few of the better-known ones. I wear overbooties and two layers of socks. I like thick slalom gloves to protect myself from the cold.

MAKING IT EASY

Once you create an opening for exercise and it becomes a habit, you'll nearly always exercise as a matter of course. That habituation can take as little as two weeks. However, you have to make it easy. The more steps you have to take, the less likely it will be that you'll fit exercise in. Here's what really works:

Exercise As You Commute

This is the best way I've found to fit in exercise every day. I made a resolution during my internship that if I could exercise every day then, I could always do it. During the winter, I'd ski the fifteen miles to the hospital. During the summer, I'd take my bike. I now live in East Harlem on Central Park. My office is about four miles away. I either blade or bike in. The round-trip gives me twenty-four minutes minimum of exercise. I then add to that by taking a detour over the George Washington Bridge and along the Palisades.

Keep Clothes at the Office

My office has long had the look of a college dormitory. I have a dozen ties hung over the edge of a bookcase. My suits are crowded onto hangers on the back of my door. There are shoes on the floor and an occasional stray sock. I've also got spare surfing shorts and T-shirts. Once a week I send the dirty clothes out and bring in some clean clothes. This way I can commute on my blades or mountain bike without carrying any extra baggage. Any homework I'll put into a knapsack.

Don't Let Travel Stop You

Travel breaks the back of the best intentioned exercise enthusiasts. For years, I used to run when I traveled. I found that fatigue from jet lag and lost sleep made it hard to run at a good enough clip for any significant period of time. About fifteen years ago I began travel-ing with my bike. It may seem cumbersome, but I found it adds a marvelous dimension to any travel experience. I've discovered the Marin headlands north of San Francisco, the small villages around Nairobi, even the dirt paths through Washington, D.C. Taking blades along is even easier. I like to check out the city ahead of time. For instance, Chicago's lakeside path, L.A.'s Santa Monica Beach path, St. Louis's riverside path, and New York's Central Park are great places to skate. A surprising number of midwestern cities have canals with blading paths next to them. My third alternative is to find a great gym. I usually substitute an evening workout for dinner.

Find the Best Gym

I belong to the World Gym across from Lincoln Center in New York. There are enough hard bodies to keep heads spinning, really terrific machines, lots of space, good music, and high energy. Find the best gym you can convenient to where you live or work.

Go for Great Scenery

I'm really particular about where I exercise. But even from New York City there are spectacular rides for cyclists along the Palisades. My favorite ride is the early morning trek from my Vermont house through Stowe to the local airport, an eighteen-mile smorgasbord of wonderful sights, sounds, and smells.

Put Music to Work

Studies show that music increases the intensity and duration of exercise. Use different tempos and kinds of music for different workouts. Try your favorite Buddy Holly classic for high-intensity days or Mozart's *Magic Flute* for a long, hard workout at an even, aggressive pace.

Tap Your Imagination

Mental imagery is an exceedingly powerful tool. Figure skaters image triple axel jumps in order to perform them. Muscle traces taken during the imaginary jump show real activity. Imagery helps you perform better. Imagery allows you to use exercise to escape the earthly bounds of daily life. Imagine you're flying an F-15 on your bike, or playing at Wimbledon when you play tennis. Kids use vivid imagery when they play. You should make every effort to revive that skill as an adult.

Wear Rose-Colored Glasses

Looking at the world through rose-colored lenses is really not a bad idea. The new sports sunglasses improve your ability to see, protect you from flying objects, and can even make industrial New Jersey, where I ride my bike in the early evenings, look pretty good. Good sunglasses also go the furthest toward giving you the look you want to intimidate those around you. They're even a good way to hide if you don't want friends to recognize you in your new Lycra one-piece racing suit.

Optically pure glasses make high-speed sports safer and easier on your eyes. Be certain that you're getting the most complete UV protection available. Otherwise, the dark lens opens your pupil up to vastly increased amounts of harmful ultraviolet light, causing early cataracts. Exposure to UV light may also worsen those with macular degeneration. Here's the American Academy of Ophthalmology's position on sunglass wear: "Wear UV absorbent sunglasses and a brimmed hat whenever you're in the sun long enough to get a suntan or a sunburn. By doing so, you reduce your risk of cataracts from the sun by 95 percent. You should shop for sunglasses that block 99 or 100 percent of all UV light. Close-fitting or wraparound lenses give you the best protection. Studies have shown that enough UV rays enter under, over, and around the sides of ordinary frames to significantly reduce the benefits of otherwise protective glasses." I've had the best luck with Revos and mixed luck with Oakleys, which can scratch easily, steam up, and rip off. Still, Oakleys have the most remarkable fit in the industry. Just be careful which one you choose.

Chapter 16

How to Recover Fast

WHEN JIMMY CONNORS PLAYED AT THE U.S. OPEN IN 1991, FANS STARED wide-eyed each time he lunged for the net, as if they were watching a fossilized dinosaur come to life. Connors amazed his fans. More often than not he made volley at net and the mad sprint back to the baseline for the ensuing lob. His performance wasn't any mystery to physiologists who study aging. Of course you can run and sprint and hit at thirty-nine just like the kids. What you can't do is recover quickly. The real experts waited for the big match against Jim Courier to see if Connors would hold up. He didn't. Courier murdered him. If he had had two days more to recover, would Connors have done better? "Let's put it this way," says Dr. William McMaster, attending physician to the U.S. swim team and a clinical professor of orthopedic surgery at the University of California, Irvine, "it's no accident that Connors is a spokesperson for Nuprin. That's the kind of thing we see all the time. He has the desire. But he simply has a tough time competing against the young guys. He can't repeat it day after day. He goes pretty far and then when it gets to the end, he drops out. The younger guys who are winning are up for the next round and they're not nearly as sore as Jimmy.

"The best way to determine how aging has affected athletes is recovery time. Swimmers train twice a day. At twenty years old they recover in six hours. At forty they take two days to recover!" The ugly fact is this: the speed of recovery can slow to a crawl as you age. It is the single most vexing problem of the aging athlete and the one that accounts for the biggest erosion of performance. "Bouncing back day after day without breaking down and withstanding the wear and tear of training is the most important problem any athlete over thirty faces," says Dr. John Wilkinson of the University of Wyoming in Laramie.

Conventional Wisdom:
Just do it.
New Paradigm:
The greatest advances in speed, endurance, and fitness come only when you learn how to recover.

WHY OLDER ATHLETES DON'T RECOVER WELL

Poor Nutrition

Many older athletes don't take advantage of the major advances in sports nutrition to recover quickly and fully.

Calorie Restriction

In a futile effort to restrict calories to stay trim and still push the limits of their performance, they do a poor job of replenishing energy stores and repairing damaged muscles.

Poor Training

"The older athlete does say he has difficulty doing the same back-to-back high-intensity workouts as he used to do. I've always believed that part of why we recover slower is that older athletes are doing less training. Even if it's a subtle difference. Even if the older athlete is even slightly less fit, he won't recover or perform as well," says Dr. Michael Pollock, professor of medicine for exercise and science and director of the Center of Exercise Science at the University of Florida in Gainesville.

Dr. Bill Evans, the director of the Noll Physiological Research Center at Pennsylvania State University, says that recovery is truly a matter of conditioning, not aging. "Ninety percent of the time, the older person doesn't put the same type of training in and it is not a surprise that their recovery isn't as good. From my standpoint, fundamentally, that's what it is. If you look at the oldest players on sports teams, they're always the best-conditioned athletes on the team. When you talk to them, they say they know what it takes to stay well conditioned, and therefore, injury free."

Dr. David Altchek, the medical director for the New York Mets and an assistant attending orthopedic surgeon at the Hospital for Special Surgery in New York, says that it's the preparation going in. The higher your level of fitness, he says, the better your recovery. As we age, it's definitely harder to achieve that level of preparticipation fitness. One factor is time. "Guys between thirty-five and forty-five years old have less time to prepare. We're not necessarily talking about professional athletes. Older athletic men starting even in their early thirties have a huge problem with recovery," says Dr. Altchek.

Stiffer Ligaments

In older athletes, the ligaments that attach muscles to bones and joints are stiffer and less elastic. Studies show that these ligaments are mechanically different from younger ligaments. They have much less give. This leads to small tears in the ligaments during intense exercise. These are called micro-injuries. "This is why the weekend athlete is still sore three days after playing hard, while a teenager can go out the next day and not be bothered by it," says Dr. William McMaster. Stiff ligaments are much more likely to suffer serious injury when pushed too hard.

Less Muscle

In an *American Journal of Pathology* article, M. J. Warhol and colleagues looked at the leg muscle of older runners under the microscope. They saw more connective and scar tissue and less muscle than in younger runners. If these older runners ran the same speed as the younger runners, what muscle they had left would have to work harder than the younger runners' muscle and would therefore require more time to recover. One important caveat. These research subjects were runners. Nonimpact sports like skating, cross-country skiing, and cycling may not result in nearly as much muscle destruction.

Declining Immune Function

Dr. Bill Evans has shown that as you grow older, immune function fades. Even the small amount of immune system decline that an athlete has in his late thirties or forties is enough to slow recovery.

Less Joint Lubrication

"If you look at a thirty-year-old baseball pitcher, you'll see that it takes him a longer time in between each pitch than a younger player. This is due to joint fluid, which we refer to as gel, which as one ages gets thickened and slows you up," says Dr. Frank H. Bassett III, professor of orthopedics and chief of the Sports Medicine Section at Duke University Medical Center.

Bad Genes

Dr. William Kraemer, director of research at the Center for Sports Medicine at Pennsylvania State University, says, "We found that recovery is very individualistic. There's probably a genetic basis, because some older athletes recover pretty well."

Anti-inflammatory Drugs

Many athletes down massive quantities of nonsteroidal anti-inflammatory drugs (NSAIDs), of which Nuprin, Advil, and Motrin are just a few. Taken before intense exercise, they will ease the pain of the workout or race. Long-term abuse of big quantities of these drugs can cause irreversible kidney damage in some susceptible athletes. Even small quantities can cause bleeding in the stomach for those sensitive to them. Dr. Bill Evans also believes that they slow the repair process: "It appears that part of the repair of muscle is mediated, in part, by prostaglandins. If you take nonsteroidal anti-inflammatories like aspirin or ibuprofen that completely block the production of prostaglandins, you may blunt the ability to repair the muscle. My general recommendation is against taking them unless you really have a joint injury or joint problem. For muscle soreness I generally am against it. If you block it beforehand with NSAIDs, you can certainly injure yourself and cause further damage. The real danger is massive overuse. A lot of athletes take these to survive. I remember a few years ago doing a study looking at muscle damage following a marathon. I was taking a muscle biopsy from one fellow who was bleeding. He told me he was taking eighteen aspirin a day. He had a groin injury and just refused to stop running."

Dr. Jim McGuire, associate dean of the Stanford Medical School, says, "If you take NSAIDs before exercise, you do push your limits further. The speculation is that you feel like you can do more, although that's only because you are numb to the pain, so you go ahead and do that extra set and you injure yourself. It's not that NSAIDs delay recovery, it's that you've injured yourself a little more. If NSAIDs are given beforehand, for whatever reason, you are vaso-constricting the kidneys and, even more, the bowels. Blood flow is not as equally distributed on an NSAID. There is a lot of ischemia that occurs and, therefore, recovery isn't as quick because the depth of injury is a little bit more."

There is a flip side. Other scientists believe that NSAIDs actually speed recovery. A prominent 1991 study published in *Medicine and Science in Sports and Exercise* demonstrated that ibuprofen taken before intense exercise can minimize soreness forty-eight hours after the exercise bout. Muscular strength was also improved over those who took no drug, even though the drug had washed out of the system by the time the testing was done.

Some preliminary studies show that anti-inflammatory drugs taken after exercise can speed recovery and allow better play sooner than would be possible without them. Priscilla Clarkson, Ph.D., a professor of exercise science at the University of Massachusetts at Amherst, says, "I'm a muscle soreness specialist, so when I talk about recovery I'm talking about recovery from strenuous effort that will induce soreness the next day. There was some concern that NSAIDs would inhibit prostaglandin release and therefore delay recovery, because that was involved in protein synthesis as well as in the pain production. We did a study to determine that, and we found that it didn't at all inhibit the recovery of strength and range of motion. We gave it after exercise."

So what's the bottom line? Routine use of NSAIDs is not a terrific idea, nor is it recommended by the FDA or the manufacturer on the package inserts. I do take them as a preventative for skiing and tennis only because excess soreness makes me clumsy and increases the likelihood I'll injure myself. While I don't advocate their use, I do find them helpful on an occasional basis. Be certain that you are not prone to their damaging effects on the kidney or stomach. If you do take NSAIDs regularly, you should have a simple kidney function test and stool test for blood loss. Do they do more good than harm? Nobody really knows.

HOW TO SPEED RECOVERY

Reload Muscle Fuel Stores Quickly

This is the best and most practical application of sports fuels. Right after a workout there is a small window of opportunity during which you can have a dramatic effect on your recovery. This narrow time window allows you to refill your muscles faster and more completely than is possible at any other time. Complete instructions are outlined in Chapter 11, "Sports Foods."

Quit While You're Ahead

Stop your workouts while you still feel fresh and strong. Even on a hard day's workout, you should feel fresh when you stop. That means you still have some fuel stores left. If not, you're making major nutritional and training errors. Daily training is not a contest to punish muscle until it's beat to a pulp and out of fuel.

Hydrate

Each of the experts I talked with agreed that poor hydration steals from any performance and greatly slows recovery. Starting at dinner the night before a match and continuing throughout the night, Jimmy Connors drinks at least the equivalent of a couple of quarts of water. If he wakes up in the night to go to the bathroom, he'll have a big glass of water then. When he wakes up, he'll have more in the morning and then back off two to three hours before the match. Only when urine has no color have you drunk enough for a major contest. Very dilute sports drinks are a great way to keep enough fluid in your system if you're losing lots of fluids at the gym, at altitude, in warm weather, or if you're overdressed. Research shows that subjects will drink more of a cool sports drink than water.

Put Out the Fire: Restore Body Buffers

Muscles produce lactic acid whenever they perform high-intensity work. The lactic acid can cause your muscles to burn and become sore and tender. Should the concentration of lactic acid become too high in the muscles, they will simply shut down. That's what happened to speed skater Dan Jansen during the 1992 Winter Olympic Games in Albertville. Dan went so hard that lactic acid buildup in his muscles simply caused them to stop working. The body has buffers that soak up lactic acid, but these buffers are spent as quickly as a fire extinguisher. Unfortunately, the most prominent buffer, bicarbonate, can take up to three days to be completely replaced. You can drink a bicarbonate solution, but more than just a little can cause cramps and diarrhea.

One popular strategy is to take phosphate pills in products like Phosfuel prior to a big event. How well phosphate pills work is a matter of some debate, although I've personally found them pretty effective. Phosphates draw lactic from muscle cells into the blood so that muscle cells can work hard without overloading on lactic acid. The best strategy is to allow two days of recovery so your body can naturally replenish your buffer stores.

Stop the Damage: Take Antioxidants After Exercise

Vigorous exercise can damage your body by generating free radicals. Likened to a madman swinging a hatchet while running wild in a china shop, free radicals may slow recovery by attacking muscle, heart, and lung tissue. A group of vitamins called antioxidants smother free radicals. For this reason, if you take antioxidants, it makes sense to take them after hard workouts. Dr. Bill Evans believes that increasing immune system function and white blood cell response greatly enhance recovery. Bill gave older exercisers 800 international units of the antioxidant vitamin E daily for two months. With the addition of vitamin E, the older athlete had the same recovery as the younger person. Unfortunately, the recommended doses of antioxidants vary wildly. There is no right dose.

The Colgan Institute in Encinitas, California, recommends individualized doses of antioxidants. Its general guidelines range from modest fitness (low number) to serious athletes (high number).

Nutrient	Daily Amount
N-acetyl cysteine	50–350 mg
L-glutathione	100–200 mg
Vitamin A (palmitate)	5,000–10,000 IU
Beta-carotene	1,000–25,000 IU
Vitamin C (as ascorbic acid)	2,000–10,000 mg
Vitamin E (as tocopherol complex)	200–800 IU
Vitamin E (as d-alpha tocopherol succinate)	400–1,200 IU
Zinc (picolinate)	10–60 mg
Selenium (selenomethionine)	200–400 mcg
Selenium (as sodium selenite)	100–200 mcg
Co-enzyme Q10	30–60 mg

Dr. Colgan has used these dosing schedules on 32,000 clients over twenty years. Only two individuals had reactions that caused them to cease taking supplements.

Dr. Charles H. Hennekens of the Harvard Medical School is concerned that antioxidants taken in supplement form may be much less useful than promoted and perhaps even dangerous. A recent study reported in the *New England Journal of Medicine* failed to show protection against lung cancer in smokers. Since most current research on the positive benefits of antioxidants comes from subjects who consumed them in foods, Dr. Colgan faults this now famous article for using extraordinarily low doses in smokers.

TRAINING

When you were twenty, you could do anything: stay up all night, drink yourself into the ground, train in a haphazard fashion, stagger to the starting line, and still emerge from the embers to race and win. It's a little different in your thirties and beyond. How do you compete and win with the kids? Intelligent training is the key, but that doesn't mean being a deadhead, a term that refers to cyclists who rack up endless miles without any thought given to strategy or quality.

Build More Muscle

"The more I study, the more I think recovery is a conditioning issue. There's more and more evidence that the type of training you do is the most important thing," says Dr. Bill Evans, who cites a Scandinavian study that looked at strength, muscle size, and molecular structure of the muscle in master athletes: weight lifters, swimmers, and runners. The study showed that the weight lifters were the only group that had the same strength, muscle size, and molecular structure as their younger counterparts. Weight lifting was the only training that maintained muscle over time.

Vary Your Weight Training

The latest research shows that bigger strength and muscle mass gains are made by varying your training between high- and low-intensity workouts. This concept is called periodization. "We simply need more time between heavy sessions. The periodization concept was developed by the former USSR and Eastern Bloc countries and in the U.S. in the late sixties. It's really the most popular training concept to prevent overtraining and therefore poor recovery," says Dr. William Kraemer of Pennsylvania State University. Periodization is planned phases of training. In the heavy phase, weights are increased and repetitions are decreased, but rest is planned before the body cries out for it. Rest and recovery comes in the form of lower weights and more repetitions. Rather than suffering unexpected ups and downs, periodization will step you up slowly with planned breaks.

Plan to Recover

Most good training programs count on seventy-two hours between intense training sessions. That's the longest it takes most men to recover. Practically speaking, that means training individual muscles hard only twice a week, whether you undertake aerobic or weight training. "The biggest problem that I see with middle age is in the concept of training. Middle-aged people believe that you do the same thing every day. This doesn't allow your body to recover in that area that you've just trained. You need to work different areas, not the same exact thing over and over," says Dr. William McMaster. If your training sessions are too intense, too close together, you won't recover. When you come to the next hard training session, your fuel stores are still empty. That increases your potential for becoming injured, stale, or overtrained.

Cross Train

Cross training is the best way to stay injury free. If you're a runner, rather than pushing hard the day after a hard day's training, skate or bike. If I want to train intensely more than twice a week, I switch sports. Since it is the muscle tissue that needs recovery, I just switch to fresh muscles I haven't spent. You can even work a different part of the same muscle by switching sports.

Here's why. Under the microscope, you can see that muscles are constructed from tiny, nearly hair-width fibers. Within a muscle you can fatigue one group of fibers and leave the fibers right next to it fresh. If you've burned your thigh muscles to a fare-thee-well by running on Monday, treat them to another hard workout on rollerblades on Tuesday. Even though blading uses the same muscles, many muscle fibers remain fresh and ready to go. The blading workout will also help clear toxic waste products out faster and massage muscle fibers that are still sore from Monday's workout. If you're a runner, cycling gets you away from the pounding that increases the hazard of injury in high-mileage training programs. When I competed in Iron Man contests, I'd cycle three hundred miles a week but run only twenty. I suffered no running injuries and still felt fast on race day.

Keep It Up

You can't have breaks in your training as you age. Older men decondition faster and take far longer to get retrained. You simply can't afford to take more than a week off.

OTHER METHODS TO SPEED RECOVERY

Go for a Massage

If you're a hard weekend warrior who is too sore to move by Sunday morning, massage is the fastest, most effective way back into action. Advocates say massage kneads out lactic acid and other metabolites. I haven't seen any convincing studies to prove how it does what it's supposed to do, but it sure works. I also respect massage therapists as excellent diagnosticians. I had terrible back and shoulder pain. A masseuse at the Top Notch Spa in Stowe, Vermont, quickly pinpointed the problem, released the tension, recommended stretching exercise and a different way to sleep. The problem disappeared in a week.

Practice Active Isolated Stretching

The most convincing single reason to stretch is to speed recovery. If muscles remain stiff when you begin your next workout, it's your best clue that you're not recovered and should back off. Try the routines in Chapter 26, "Building Elastic Muscle." I've found I can ride hard day in and day out on a fitness vacation by employing them.

Rest Longer Than You Think You Need

Recovery from strenuous, fatiguing exercise requires more time than most athletes think. Research suggests that even when muscle fuel

stores are completely refilled, the muscles' ability to function, to produce power, is still impaired. The probable reason is the extra time
required for damaged muscle to repair itself, which is longer than it
takes for muscles to refuel. Even after seven days on a high-
carbohydrate diet, runners recovering from a marathon who continued to train, even at their own pace, did not recover full muscle
function. Rest doesn't mean no workout. It simply means exercising
at a lower intensity until you are fully recovered. There is no bigger
mistake athletes over thirty make than eliminating the proper recovery period.

SLEEP

With age, we get less and less deep sleep. A third of children's sleep
is deep. At age fifty, only 20 percent of the night is spent in deep
sleep. Return to a night of deep sleep and you will return to your
youth. A lack of sleep can slowly destroy your personality, your physical stamina, and your ability to get any meaningful work done. Dr.
Quentin Regestein, director of the Sleep Clinic at the Brigham and
Women's Hospital in Boston, says, "Sleep is a kind of barometer for
your health in general. Everything affects your sleep, so you want
everything at its most optimal."

Treat sleep with the same veneration as you would physical or
mental preparation for sport or work, and you will become a new
person. Each one of us requires a fixed amount of sleep. Cheat the
sandman and you'll pay with your life. Chronic lack of sleep reduces
your life expectancy. Lack of sleep is one of the leading causes of loss
of life from industrial and automobile accidents. The few accidents
I've had in recent years were all due to a lack of sleep. The hours
you gain from giving up sleep, you'll likely lose to colds, flus, and
sore throats, because a lack of sleep dampens the immune system as
well. Worst of all, poor sleep will make you old — fast! Dr. Joyce
Walsleben, director of the Sleep Disorder Center at New York University, says, "In my opinion, we're all pretty sleep deprived. It's been
shown that you should have between six and ten hours of sleep per

night. People who sleep less than six hours or more than ten hours have a higher mortality rate."

When I first began working in early morning television, I made a remarkable discovery. I could get up at 5 A.M. all right, but I couldn't function. The anchor would ask me a question, and I would delay long enough for my brain to fire a few sorry circuits. By the time that happened, the anchor had a nearly panicked look on her face. I resolved to go to bed earlier so I could better feign alertness. But going to bed early didn't help. I'd wrestle around for hours trying to make myself go to sleep with little success. I consulted Chuck Czeisler, M.D., a sleep expert at Harvard Medical School. He reassured me that all I lacked was good sleep hygiene. Sleep hygiene? You mean like taking a shower before bedtime? I asked. He calmly explained that was not exactly what he meant. A huge number of Americans sleep poorly because they prepare to sleep poorly, he said. I left with a set of suggestions that I followed to the letter. Within weeks, I became bright and perky in the morning and saved my fledgling career. If you're sleepy during the day and not able to stay awake when driving or at meetings, it may not be that you're just getting older. You need to consider your sleep as a culprit.

Dr. Walsleben emphasizes the importance of reinforcing your body as opposed to breaking it down. "Men between the ages of thirty-five and fifty-five typically don't care for themselves well. They work too hard, they're always running, and, in general, don't allow enough hours for sleep," she observes. Here are the key steps to a great night's sleep.

Don't Oversleep

A precisely calibrated body clock is your best single guarantee of high-quality sleep. Body clocks time all bodily functions. During a given twenty-four-hour period, there are peaks and troughs for everything from temperature, psychological test performance, and alertness to hormone levels. All of these fluctuate predictably. For example, cortisone, the stress hormone, is highest for most people at

8:00 A.M. and lowest at midnight. Dr. Walsleben says, "Meals at regular times and all activities, like exercising, at predictable times will strengthen the wake system to be awake when you want to be and help calm you down when it's time for the sleep system."

The best way to set your body clock in stone is to wake up every day at the same time. That includes weekends. Every extra hour you sleep requires a full twenty-four hours to reset. If you get up at 7 A.M. weekdays and 10 A.M. Sunday, it'll be Wednesday before your body is back on track. That's why Mondays usually feel so rough. If the body is set on one activity cycle and a different sleep/wake cycle, you'll be in a state of jet lag. "It's vital to regularize," says Dr. Walsleben. If you party hard and late, get up at your regular time, even if you have to nap later. You'll be groggier and pay for it days later if you sleep in. "You don't necessarily have to go to sleep at the same time every night. It's more important to wake up every day at the same time. But if you get up every day at the same time, you'll eventually end up going to sleep at the same time," says Dr. Regestein.

No Nervous System Acting Drugs Before Sleep

"At the end of a long day, men want to calm down. Many choose drugs or alcohol, which automatically changes the architecture of sleep. We have normal highs and lows of sleep, and drugs of any sort disrupt those natural occurrences," says Dr. Walsleben. Here are the biggest villains:

- alcohol
- nicotine
- nasal decongestants
- sleeping pills
- diet pills
- high-blood-pressure medications
- bronchodilators
- cortisone
- caffeine

In most men, caffeine has a very long duration of action, from twelve to twenty hours, so the coffee you have with lunch can destroy your sleep that night. This response is quite individual. Some men can drink a cup right before they go to bed and sleep just fine. Others can't drink coffee after noon or else they won't get to sleep until two or three in the morning. If you think coffee is the problem, try to keep moving your cup or two of coffee back an hour until your sleep isn't affected by it. You may be one of those people who shouldn't be drinking coffee at all.

No Alcohol Before Sleep

Even if you don't recognize the phenomenon, a late night drink will retard the presence of dream sleep. You will miss out on it in the beginning of your sleep and never fully make up for it. Toward the morning hours, your body will shift into a very intense dream sleep, causing your blood pressure and temperature to fluctuate, and your heart may beat abnormally. If you're overweight or have a bad heart, this more intense dream state can harm you. Alcohol, says Dr. Regestein, may first act as a sedative, but it later disturbs sleep by stimulating production of adrenaline-like neurotransmitters, interfering with breathing and increasing the need to urinate. Even alcoholics who quit continue to suffer lighter and more fragmented sleep than normal.

No Smoking

Smoking interferes with the quality of your sleep. A study in England in 1980 found that the more you smoke, the less you sleep. Researchers found that smoking one pack a day reduced sleeping by nearly a half hour at night. There is good news if you quit. Dr. Constantine Soldatos, formerly of the University of Pennsylvania, discovered that after only one week after quitting, patients began to sleep better. Dr. Regestein adds, "Many patients who need help regarding sleep are smokers."

Exercise — But Not Before Bed

The higher your metabolic rate, the deeper your sleep. If you have a high metabolic rate, you'll sleep like a baby. The bad news is that, as you age, metabolic rate drops, causing a sharp deterioration in sleep. A sedentary thirty-year-old gets half of the highest-quality stage 4 sleep that a twenty-year-old does. I call this an old-getting-older phenomenon. I look at people my own age who are gray and old. They've entered into a vicious cycle. By undertaking a sedentary lifestyle they never get quality sleep. They make up for the lack of well-being with food, alcohol, caffeine, even drugs and cigarettes, and rapidly accelerate the cycle of aging. However, by using exercise as their drug of choice, they can crank back the years. A sedentary middle-aged male in an exercise program can increase his metabolic rate within six weeks.

Make Your Bedroom a Vault

Sleep experts are astounded by the amount of noise men unconsciously put up with as they try to sleep. You may be able to fall asleep when you're exhausted, but those nights you settle in for a full eight hours will be tough if your neighbor's boombox or your kid's electric guitar is cranked up to warp sound. When we bought an apartment five years ago, my first concern was bedroom noise. Since a noisy bedroom is so debilitating to your sleep and therefore to your overall ability to concentrate during the day or get a decent workout, it should be one of the first priorities in selecting where you sleep. When I select a hotel room, I'll ask for a corner room away from the elevators. Some men need a level of ambient background noise such as traffic, a river flowing, or ocean roar or they can't sleep. You can bring that on the road with you as a white noise generator.

Sleep on an Empty Stomach

My mother always said half the world went to bed hungry. Well at least half the world now has a chance of getting a good night's sleep. Here's why: a big meal before bedtime is a surefire way to spend the night staring at the ceiling. The sheer volume of food can push its way back up into your esophagus. Stomach acid is very strong stuff and can cause a good deal of pain. Your stomach can handle it, but your esophagus can't. Too much roughage can also cause a poor night's sleep by keeping your intestines at work, so avoid too much steak, bran, and raw vegetables at dinnertime.

Establish a Routine

Intense, high-functioning men who learn fast and are scrupulously introspective get into bed at night and can't turn it off. They are easily aroused by an argument or an annoying phone call. They are unable to make the transition into sleep. Men like this and all men experiencing stress need a relaxing evening routine with a predictable train of rituals: regular dinnertime, dry the dishes, play with the kids, read a book, brush teeth, get into bed, and turn out the light.

Put Your Worries On Hold

Dr. Walsleben has found a successful way for her patients to ease their way into sleep time. Set an afternoon time to consolidate worries on a piece of paper. Write down the key problem items and solutions. Keep it in your pocket. Take it to bed and fold it up and put it on your bedtable. Realize that it will be there in the morning and you don't have to ruminate about it throughout the night.

Switch On Visual Imagery

I've found imaging a flawless technique for falling asleep or getting back to sleep. I used to wake at 4 A.M. and begin to ruminate about a variety of anxiety-producing events. Now if I wake up in the wee hours or can't get to sleep, I switch to visual imagery. Although the cartoon version of this is counting sheep, I'll image ski turns or tennis shots and practice them in my mind until I fall asleep. Within minutes, I'm out like a light. You may want to image sound as well. If you're imaging a windsurfing lesson, listen to the slow rhythm of the waves. If you can't do this well on your own in the beginning, there are audiotapes that will put you in a pleasant imaginary situation and walk you through it.

Know Your Sleeping Pattern

There really are morning people and night people. Morning people sleep lighter and lighter as the night turns into morning so that they veritably pop out of bed. Evening people sleep deeper and deeper as the night turns into morning. By 6 A.M., they're really into deep sleep. They drag themselves out of bed and gradually recover during the day. They're most productive and creative at evening. These aren't disorders, they're reality.

Have Sex

Although little research among sleep experts has been done on sex, Dr. Regestein believes that, like a hot bath or anything else that reduces tension, it will help.

Follow a Checklist

Experts suggest a checklist to ensure that all these elements are optimal for you.

- Temperature. Too warm and you'll wake up in the wee hours. Above 75 to 80 degrees may interfere with sleep. However, the correct temperature does depend on how you were brought up. Arabs freeze in anything below 70 degrees. You're the best measure of too hot, not the thermostat. If you feel too hot, it's too hot.
- Mattress comfort. Too soft and you'll wake up with a backache.
- Light. The less the better.
- Activity of bed partner. Don't feel you're being insensitive if your bedmate keeps you up. If they do, take action! When my wife snores, I sleep on the floor in my son's room. "I'm also a big promoter of separate beds if one partner is keeping the other awake," says Dr. Walsleben.

PLAY SPORTS

Chapter 17

Alpine Skiing

THE VIEW FROM THE START HOUSE OF THE MEN'S DOWNHILL AT Val d'Isère looks down through a rock chute better suited to an elevator shaft than a ski run. Franz Klammer invited me to ski the course with him for a *CBS This Morning* piece on the aerobic benefits of ski racing. During a slow-speed examination of the course, Franz recounted the grim injuries that had befallen lesser racers at each major turn or transition. We took a second, more serious run. With 223 cm Rossignol Downhills strapped to my feet, I felt as if I had been dropped out of an airplane each time the earth fell away. Franz and I tucked to the bottom. In the race finish area I looked at my heart-rate monitor. Wow! 176! I showed Franz and remarked that Alpine skiing really was a wonderful aerobic sport. "That's higher than most aerobic sports." Franz looked at me and said, "Bob, your heart rate is one seventy-six because you're scared."

Scared or not, Alpine skiers get a terrific workout. Skiing builds great aerobic power and tremendous muscular strength and explosiveness. Twenty years ago only great skiers got a great workout, because skiing required such huge amounts of baseline conditioning. Now elegant techniques, cutting-edge technology, and rapid talent advancement have opened up the universe of world-class skiing to the weekend athlete.

Conventional Wisdom:
Skiing is recreation, like bowling.
New Paradigm:
Skiing is a spectacular workout.

WHY YOU SHOULD CONSIDER ATHLETIC SKIING

It's a Fast, Efficient Workout

Skiing has been transformed from an all-day outing into a two- to three-hour workout. In the old days you'd have a good day if you got twelve to fifteen runs from 8 A.M. to 4 P.M. The lifts were slow. Ungroomed slopes meant you'd have to pick your way down. Equipment made it difficult to ski far without fatigue. Now lifts shoot you to the top of a big mountain in seven minutes. Super grooming gives you long, continuous leg-burning runs. In three hours of hard skiing you're done, ready to go on to the next sport or back to your family responsibilities.

Skiing Is a Transformed Sport

Skiing is a much different sport than it was ten years ago. The technology in today's skis, boots, and bindings is so advanced that you can ski far better, cleaner turns with greater ease and far fewer broken bones. Boots are really comfortable and warm. Skis are easier to turn and hold on the hardest ice. Twenty years ago very few men could ski at 50 mph safely and under control. Now the average man with the right terrain and equipment can ski powerfully, fast, and safely thanks to technology and new trail-grooming equipment.

Great Skiing Is Closer Than Aspen

You might not consider Alpine skiing as regular fitness activity because so much of the skiing public has moved to a once-a-year western holiday. If you live out West and live near a ski area, you can stop reading right here, but if you live in the Northeast, the far West, or the upper Midwest, reconsider Alpine skiing as a terrific way to stay in shape during the cold months and beat the winter blues. What's changed? Go out to a bare ski hill in early winter. Then watch a good snow-making crew turn on its guns. In three days that hill can be covered to perfection. Snow grooming has reached such an advanced state that you'll find the hill prepped like a race course with not a rock showing or piece of ice left, making for terrific ski conditions all winter long. My family skis Stowe, Vermont, from Thanksgiving to Easter. There's never a weekend that you can't get a great workout. With high-speed lifts and bottom-to-top service, skiers get much more skiing in three hours at Stowe than in a whole day at Vail or Aspen.

Skiing Is an Athlete Builder

Weekend skiing motivates you to keep fit during the week in ski-specific activities such as Stairmasters, blading, and biking. Skiing builds power, balance, concentration, coordination plus aerobic power. Skiing will keep you young. "I never met a serious skier who had a midlife crisis" is the chant of the avid skier.

SPORTS-IMPROVEMENT TECHNOLOGY

BOOTS

The boot is the most critical piece of ski equipment. Dave Bertoni, product information manager of Salomon North America, says, "In my opinion, skiers are hampered most by an ill-fitting boot and one that doesn't support them in the right angle. I would go as far as to say that most ski instructors have the same problem. Without a good fit, the chances that they're going to have an enjoyable or successful experience are not good." The right boot, fitted correctly, can make you a great skier overnight. The wrong boot or fit will sap any athleticism you bring to the sport.

Rear-entry boots are a great example of what can go wrong. Most of them hold skiers rigidly upright where they cannot press forward to ski properly. But even the right boot can detract from your performance. A survey conducted by Burke Mountain Ski Academy founder and champion coach Warren Witherell shows that "only 10 percent of all skiers, when buckled in rigid boots, have ideal skeletal alignment." That means that 90 percent of skiers are technically handicapped and simply won't be able to ski anywhere near their potential.

I bought Witherell's book *The Athletic Skier* and quickly determined that I, too, had a problem. My knee wouldn't stay pointed in toward the hill. When I did get it in to carve a turn, my knee wobbled in and out of the turn. With book in hand, I went to my local boot fitter in Stowe. José shook his head. "You're two degrees to the outside." Gee, two degrees, that didn't seem like much. But José quickly explained that all my technical errors were due to my boots. Wow. A poor workman *can* blame his tools!

Here are the problems boot technicians most commonly find in men:

Bowleg. You needn't actually have bowlegs to have this condition. Your lower leg simply needs to bow out of your boot, which was exactly my problem. I was two degrees to the outside of centerline. I should have been two degrees inside centerline for edge quickness.

Knock-knee. It's a real advantage in skiing to be slightly knock-kneed because you stand naturally on your inside edge. But past two degrees and your skiing will suffer badly. Your skis will slide and skid, and the ski will turn too slowly. Because you can't hold an edge, you won't be fast or athletic. Those skiers who are excessively knock-kneed can be corrected back toward a more neutral stance by adding one or more degrees to the outside edge of the boot.

Combination. You'll have one knee pointed in and the other pointed out, leading to any of the above-mentioned errors, depending on the direction of the turn. With perfect alignment you can expect to be relaxed and free of fatigue. You will naturally carve a turn and be able to use fully all your natural agility, quickness, and explosiveness. You'll also avoid skidded turns and begin to look like a real pro. These errors are easily corrected by any good boot fitter. Many will perform this service as part of the price of the boot. Here are the steps they will take to correct your alignment.

Many skiers' feet tend to collapse toward the inside or outside of the turn, making the skis wobble. These alignment problems and many others in the structure of the foot are best fixed with a custom footbed. While you stand with your knees bent and your legs properly aligned in the correct position for skiing, a heated footbed is placed under your feet. Once this has cooled and been trimmed and fitted into your boot, it supports your foot so that it won't collapse in the wrong direction when all the considerable forces of skiing are applied to your foot.

You can correct much of the actual bowlegged or knock-kneed error by moving the upper part of the boot shell in or out. If this doesn't correct the error fully, the sole of the boot can be ground down on the inside or outside to further correct any errors. Salomon has a cantable sole. You can change the angle of the boot by changing the sole pads on the bottom.

If you still are not completely corrected, you can apply cants to the ski itself. For fast, wide-radius skiing, you will want to be no more than two degrees to the inside. For rapid gate-slalom racing, you can go as much as four degrees to the inside. Purists believe that canting should be done at the level of the ski, not the boot. The rationale is that most boot canting is just changing the upper cuff, not the lower boot, which is what really counts.

When you're all finished, be certain that you are equally strong on your inside and outside edges. If you can't ski onto your outside edges, you may be overcanted. My ski instructor pointed this out, and I had my boot fitter add a heel lift to cant me back to the outside.

In racing boots, stiffness is still the name of the game. Alberto Tomba will stick his boots in ice before a race to get them maximally stiff. But be warned, leading U.S. ski coach Dave Merriam finds most skiers are in boots that are too stiff. New boots can vary the stiffness of the forward and the sideways flex. You may want a very soft forward flex but a very stiff side flex to get quickly from edge to edge. Tecnica's TNT is one example of these new versatile boots.

For all but World Cup racers, boots now rate very high on the comfort scale. Independent heating systems also keep your feet toasty warm well below zero. I've had good luck with Heatronics when the battery stayed on the boot. Batteries tend to get dinged by chairlifts and end up lost in the snow. When your battery is still attached to the boot, you'll find it warm even at zero degrees.

PLATFORMS

Look at a racer's boots. Underneath them you'll see platforms that lift the boot off the ski. They range from simple lifters and spacers to expensive brand-name products such as the Derby Flex, Salomon's new suspension binding, and Alan Trimble's PB Turbo floater. Here's what they do:

The first benefit of the platform is as a vibration filter. If you don't have a platform to absorb vibration, your legs become the filter. As a result, your muscles will tire out faster trying to keep the ski stable.

An elevated boot increases the leverage you have over a ski so that it is easier to put on its edge. This is most useful for GS, Super G, and downhill racing. Raising the binding is done in part out of necessity. The more radical side-cut skis are narrower than the ski boot. With radical angulation, racers suffer "boot out," that is, the boot hits the snow and knocks the ski off its carve. Elevated bindings give you a bigger footprint on the ski. Advocates liken it to skiing on a two-foot-long ski. An elevated boot lets you ski "big foots" like Atomic's Heli-Guide on hard snow.

Some bindings allow you to change the stiffness of the ski by a flip of a lever on the front of the binding. Number one is for slow turns, since it allows the ski's full flex to come into play. The highest setting, three, stiffens the ski, so it holds better at high speed without as much work on the part of the skier. This feature gives you three skis in one.

Even at the highest levels of international competition, racers get away with shorter skis by using platforms for stability.

If you have a ski that's built for slower speeds and shorter radius turns and want to make it more lively, use a dynamic platform.

BINDINGS

New binding technology accounts for a radical reduction in lower-leg ski injuries, according to a study conducted by the president of Vermont Safety Research Carl Ettlinger; University of Vermont professor of orthopedics and rehabilitation Dr. Robert Johnson; and Dr. Jasper Shealy, chairman of the industrial engineering department at Rochester Institute of Technology. In fact, the Johnson study shows that broken legs, ankle sprains, and ankle fractures were each reduced 90 percent. Be sure to look for bindings with upward toe release. Have a certified binding technician check your bindings each year. Top racers make the costly error of outguessing the manufacturer and setting bindings so they just can't come out. If you've seen the Olympic or World Cup coverage, you may have witnessed spectacular crashes where the skis never come off. At 90 mph there is a tiny line between safe and sorry. For recreational skiers, there is a huge margin for error if your bindings are set correctly. With better damping and less vibration, there is no reason to have super-high binding settings. You can ski a downhill racing ski at 70 mph on a conventional recreational setting without fear of coming out.

SKIS

When I lived in Austria during 1968, the Kneissl White Star RSE was the hottest ski to buy. It was stiff enough to use as river-crossing pontoons for standard-issue Warsaw Pact tanks, and took the strength of a bull to turn. One day at the Axamer-Lizum ski area, I met an American woman with brand-new Head 360 skis. I looked down at them in disdain. What a wimp! Cheater skis! But then I saw how easily she skied. That was my first introduction to sports-improvement technology: skis designed to make better skiers.

Current technology has come a long way. Modern skis can slip and slide enough to make skiing easy, even on double black diamond slopes. However, you'll see only one skier in a hundred who skis properly, because it's so much more natural to slide a ski than carve it. The wrong ski forces many men to ski badly. The right ski will coax you into carving nice round perfect GS turns or quick sharp J turns, pounding through the bumps or blasting through bottomless powder every time. Buy the ski for the way you want to ski. The technology is here today so that the ski almost teaches you. Here are the key ingredients.

Radical side cuts. Ski manufacturers are racing to get new skis to market that have very deep side cuts. K2 Corporation in Vashon, Washington, was the first to market with its "deep dish" Race GS Ski. This ski has fat tips and tails with a very narrow hourglass middle. It has a great combination of a deep side cut with excellent torsion control. That means the ski won't twist at high speed, allowing much tighter, higher-speed turns with better edge grip. This has led to dramatic improvements for both World Cup racers and recreational skiers. Now most skiers can get a ski onto a carving edge and keep it there. If you have not found success carving turns, this new geometry will make an enormous difference. Even at high speed, the deep, stable carve makes you feel secure.

Shorter length. It's no secret among beginning skiers that shorter skis are easier to turn and maneuver. Better skiers have turned up their noses at short skis, but World Cup racers don't. Where racers used to ski slalom on 207 cm skis, they now use 201 cm skis. Where GS was raced on 215s, they now use 204s. Why? New materials are so strong that they can create the stability and speed of a much longer ski in a short ski. Shorter skis combine the best of great maneuverability with high speed. If you skid your turns, you'll think a longer ski is better because you have more edge to scrape on the snow. But if you're going for a pure carve, then what you really want is a deep side cut and lots of stability, because you're going to go like blazes. Dave Merriam of the Stowe Mountain Resort Ski School often finds that "men buy skis that are over their head." A very long ski has to be skidded to keep it at a reasonable speed. If you are able to carve your turns with very little skidding, you'll go surprisingly fast on a short ski.

Less vibration. The first generation of light skis came at a terrible price: bone-shaking, teeth-chattering vibration. Now ski engineers can decrease edge-grip vibration so skis don't chatter on the ice and decrease high-speed chatter as well. That's tougher than it sounds. Too much vibration damping and the skis feel dead; too little and you'll need a good dentist. Wood decreases vibration over the length of the ski for downhill and super GS skis. Discrete damping is accomplished by placing higher-tech materials like urethane in specific areas of the ski to achieve maximum damping on the parts of the ski most prone to chatter and to isolate the ski from the high-speed chatter created by icy conditions. Many high-tech GS skis still use metal tops so that they remain predictable, stable, and quiet.

More stability. Higher swing weight means a more stable ski at speed, just as a heavier car is more comfortable at higher speeds. Researchers have determined that the entire ski need not be heavy, there just needs to be more weight at the tip of the ski. Salomon uses a tip protector to put a little weight at the end of the ski for greater stability. This actually works pretty well. Long, heavy skis used to be the only kind that could go fast and remain stable. Now World Cup downhill champions can race on a 210 cm ski instead of a 223.

The monocoque. Marketed as the design revolution of the 1990s, the monocoque concentrates pressure on the ski's edges so that less effort is required to hold the ski on ice. The monocoque design allows the skier to leverage the ski more easily to bite into ice with less effort for more edge grip. Skier effort is decreased as much as 18 percent. Mike Bisner, former vice president in charge of operations and marketing for the Boston-based Ski Market, says that "it effectively cuts through ice like a knife." Monocoque means "one shell." You can understand the monocoque system by imagining a rowboat turned upside down. Dave Bertoni, Salomon's product information manager, says, "If you were to stand on the top of the rowboat, all the energy goes to the rails. Our ski structure is a self-carrying, or load-bearing, inverted U. All the energy goes right to the ski edges. This gives you a lot more energy or edge grip." But beware the fake monocoque. Jim Vandergrift, director of research and development for K2 Corporation, told me that many companies just put new graphics and a new top on the ski so it looks like a monocoque when in fact it's a traditional ski underneath — sort of like putting a Ferrari body on a Volkswagen chassis.

Viselike edge grip. Skier opinion surveys have consistently shown that edge grip comes out on top as a requirement for a good ski. The monocoque is the newest anti-ice design in that it transfers all the available force to the ski's edges so that they slice through ice and hard pack. K2 uses a high-tech braided weave to increase edge grip.

Easy turning. When I tested skis in preparation for writing this book, I found a striking difference in the speed with which I could initiate a turn. By taking weight out of the front of the skis, manufacturers have created a ski that turns much faster. The reason is simple physics. Tip and tail weight are the farthest from your boot. The farther the weight is from your boot, the more energy it requires to turn. To convince yourself of that, just swivel your ski while riding a chairlift. The momentum built up by the weight at the ends of the ski takes a fair amount of force to counteract even when the ski is not on snow. It's not because the skis weigh a lot, it's because of the distance that the weight is from your foot. By taking weight out of the tips and tails of the skis, they become much easier to turn. Today's GS skis turn as quickly as the slalom skis of two to three years ago.

Softer skis. A softer overall flex makes skis much easier to turn. Softer skis allow a rounder arc to the ski, which enhances the carving capability. Engineers still make skis torsionally rigid so that they don't twist and lose their bite on ice, but also build in a soft midsection that concentrates force under the foot, producing skis that can turn easily yet hold like razors on ice.

Designer flex. Technology really comes to the fore in the flex designs of skis. In the old days a ski was either stiff or soft because it was made from stiff or soft materials. Now any part of a ski can be made stiff or soft so that it can be customized for the best possible performance. Jim Vandergrift, of K2 Corporation, says, "One of the things that we've been able to do since the days of all-wooden skis is that we have composite technology. You can tailor the longitudinal flex with the torsional flex. A ski basically has a torsional property — an ability to resist twist — and a longitudinal flex, which is its ability to resist bending. We've been able to decrease the flex while maintaining torsion. This way you can hold well on ice or hard-packed snow." What kinds of flex patterns should you look for? Here are some different principles.

- **Moguls skis.** These are stiffer in the back, so bump skiers can quickly get off the back of the ski at the end of the turn. This is combined with a deep side cut for the short turns between moguls.
- **High-speed stable skis.** These are stiffer overall and give up forgiveness for speed.
- **Ice skis.** These are designed with greater resistance to twisting, especially under the foot. Skis with high "torque" or resistance to twisting at the ends can be very unforgiving skis in any conditions.
- **J-turn skis.** The soft tip and forebody help you get the ski into the turn quickly, and the stiff tail helps you get out of the turn quickly.
- **Powder skis.** Softer torsion throughout the body makes the ski ideal for skiing on powder.

Extreme width. This is the biggest revolution in skis. Fat-boy skis make a bigger footprint on the snow because they are wider. This gives them more surface area on which to float to the top of powder snow while allowing them to be shorter for greater maneuverability. Saloman's newly appointed Director of Winter Sports Marketing Mike Bisner points out that their greatest forte is in crud where normal skis sink and become very difficult to turn.

"Typically, eastern skiers travel to the back bowls of Vail expecting bottomless powder. Instead they find day-old, warmed-over heavy snow that they can't ski to save their lives. They changed to Bigfoots, which allowed them to easily ski through difficult conditions." The fat-boy skis allow intermediate skiers to ski deep, bottomless powder. Men who never considered Canadian helicopter skiing now have the chance. "The fatigue factor is just amazing. You can spend thirty percent less energy skiing. Intermediates come out to the Bugaboos and outski the experts on fat boys," says Mike Bisner. If you want a great ski for the spring and for mashed potato snow and still want to ski western powder, consider the skis that have less extreme width. Atomic Heli-Guides are midwidth between fat-boy and regular skis. They have the side cut to ski on groomed snow. For advanced skiers who don't need the superfloat of the very wide skis, the Heli-Guides are a good junk-snow, crud, and powder ski. I love them for all-out cruising, because they have the running surface and stability of a downhill with the turning radius of a short GS ski. I believe many skiers will turn to these midwidth skis for an all-round ski. Atomic has three side cuts this year for the Heli-Guide. The Performer by S Ski has a wild radical side cut with the tip and tail of a fat boy but the skinny waist of a slalom ski. Ted Grayson, an instructor at Mount Mansfield in Stowe, Vermont, who borrowed mine, called it the best carving ski of all time.

Better ski tuning. How skis are tuned makes a tremendous difference in how you ski on them. Warren Witherell believes that the whole ski should be sharpened tip to tail so the entire carving surface of the ski is available. Many ski-tuning services will dull the tip and tail for skiers who swivel, slide, and pivot their skis. Warren says it's as if they've cut off the tips and tails of the skis and left you to pivot on the middle of the ski, in essence eliminating the key performance qualities of the ski. Many shops will bevel the edge to cant the ski but this too detunes the ski. Any canting should be done in the boot or on the top of the ski, not on the edges. Ben Gaylord of the Vail Race Department in Vail, Colorado, sharpens the entire length of the ski but will dull some of the tip until the ski comes around into a good turn. He also recommends having the edge sharpened at less than 90 degrees so that you have a razor-sharp edge. How are skis best tuned? Warren Witherell says skis should be dead flat to perform best. Doug Adams of Today's Edge in Stowe, Vermont, who tunes skis for many major races and equipment tests, uses incredibly high-tech machines to pattern the bottom of the ski. Locals swear they have a brand-new ski when they leave Doug's shop. Don't give your skis to a hack!

Weight. Carbon fiber, Kevlar, and aerospace alloys make skis extremely light while still retaining high levels of durability. There really isn't a need for a heavy ski unless you are racing Super G or downhill. Wood is used as a damping material to ease vibration and works very effectively, but acrylics lighten the weight considerably as an alternate way of damping vibration.

Light skis aren't better skis unless the weight is properly distributed. If you have extremely light tips and tails, your ski will be highly unstable. Salomon, king of lightweight skis, adds weight to the outside of the ski, near the tip, tail, and edges for added stability. Dave Bertoni of Salomon says, "We keep the ski very light on the inside and keep the weight on the outside. This puts any weight right on the snow. If there are any shocks from the side, you have mass on the snow which keeps the ski directionally stable."

Variable designer sidewalls. Look at a ski from twenty years ago and you'll see a tall, vertical sidewall that continues the full length of the ski. On newer high-tech skis, the sidewall is vertical underneath your foot and becomes increasingly sloped toward the tip and the tail of the ski. There are two benefits: improved edge grip and the ability to enter into the beginning phase of a turn more easily.

Faster running surface. Structuring the bases of Alpine skis has become a science. Different patterns are laid in for varying snow conditions and temperatures. Base materials make or break a ski's success. The best technology allows maximum speed and control. Salomon's Dave Bertoni says, "One of the most important things in snow skiing is the quality of the finish of the bottom of the ski. If your edges aren't sharp, if they're not smooth, if the bottom isn't perfectly ninety degrees, the ski simply doesn't perform well. Ninety-nine percent of the skiers in the world ski with their skis in really crappy condition. Even ski instructors' skis are covered with pockmarks on the bottom, rough spots and scratches on the edges. The skis belonging to a World Cup skier are just the opposite: they are absolutely perfect every day they ski."

Testing Skis

Make sure you're anatomically aligned before you test skis, otherwise it's not a fair test of the ski. Try the skis you think you'll like best early in the morning when they are really well tuned. Ask if their tips and tails have been blunted for ease of turning. Many companies do this so you'll like the ski's ease of turning. But if you're on ice, be ready to sled! I tried skis at Stowe demo day. It was the first real boilerplate day in years because of rain the night before. It was the truest test of what would carve and what would not. Some skis just left you naked out there, going sideways on edge faster than down-hills going tips first. Early-season demo days are a good way to get a broad range of skiing experiences. Even if you're not going to buy, you'll learn lots about skiing from the different ways the skis turn. By early afternoon on demo days, most skis look like they've been used to slide down a rock pile. Only the most fastidious reps will keep their skis tuned. For a true test, before you buy, pay the $20 most areas ask to demo some highly tuned, well-prepped skis to see if you really like them.

High-tech skis allow you to carve turns easily while maintaining tremendous stability and excellent edge grip. This was not available to the recreational skier or even World Cup skier a few years ago. You can carve a ski with far greater ease and elegance than you could ever imagine without the need for the enormous strength of a world-class racer. As Warren Witherell says, "Virtually all ski manufacturers are working to make skis that carve rather than skid and make skiing easier and more graceful. From our perspective, the designers have produced extraordinary skis, but too few skiers have learned how to use them." That's why sports-improvement technology and getting good fast go hand in hand.

ACCESSORIES

Poles. The hot new poles are very thin and have much more give than the old aluminum poles. I like them because you can pole hard without hurting your elbow. They're analogous to good cross-country skating poles. The quick-release straps will spare you many a skier's thumb. Goode was the highest-rated pole by ski magazines for the 1994 season.

Goggles. There's still no perfect goggle. I bought the Smith goggle with blowers. On the coldest subzero days, the blower actually freezes moisture that's trapped inside on the goggle, making it impossible to ski. Until someone makes a wire-heated glass, skiers will remain blind in certain situations.

GETTING GOOD FAST

Skiing is the quintessential "Don't teach me I'm great" sport. There is more ego involved in the way we ski than in the way we do almost anything else. Many of us have a picture in our mind's eye of our skiing form. It looks just like a race picture of A. J. Kitt gunning through a tight turn at 90 mph on the Olympic downhill. Those of us who have suffered the ignominy of a videotape session will find that the way we think we look has no relation to our actual form. But even if you do have flawless form, skiing technique has drastically changed in just the last several years since rapid-gate slalom and tight-gate GS have hit the World Cup circuit.

New techniques mean that you can ski very fast with tremendous power, control, and safety. Senior racing clinics have taught older men to skid their skis because they don't have the power to hold an edge. The new "railroad turn" puts huge amounts of pressure on your frame, sparing your muscle. Since weight is distributed between two skis, this decreases the effort even more. Mastering the railroad turn means that you'll be a fast, powerful skier to a ripe old age. Curiously, the railroad turn was discovered when a ski school instructor asked a simple question: How is it that kids can ski all day long without getting tired? The answer was that they hang lots of pressure on their frame and distribute the weight between two skis. The new technique is fast, powerful, and gives you a huge safety edge because of enormous control. I watch my six-year-old make railroad turns. He has both skis weighted. With the enormous hip flexibility that kids have, he hangs his hips radically into the inside of the turn with his skis parallel and widely spaced like railroad tracks. His skis are deeply set into the snow, so they can't do anything but carve a spectacular turn. From that position he can lean forward to shorten the radius of the turn.

Skiing is also a curious sport because there is no score or handicapping system. "Golf and tennis have objective scores, and with those scores a real impetus to get better. Most skiers think their handicap is in the single digits: most of them would be surprised to find that they're in the high teens," says John Douglas, president of Atomic Skis in Amherst, New Hampshire. The result is a large number of terminal intermediates. If you want to take up skiing or get remarkably better quickly, here's what to do.

Create an Image

The books *World Cup Skiing* and Warren Witherell's *The Athletic Skier* have excellent still pictures of skiing. Since skiers move in so many different planes, it's tough to analyze motion pictures, so try to get a sense of where every body part is at different points in the turn from still pictures. Then try to fill in the blanks between these still photos by videotaping ski races or bump contests on TV and playing them back at slow speed. If you don't have a slow-motion device on your VCR, hit the pause button and study where each body part is at each point in time. Race footage is good because you can see each part of the turn in relation to the gate.

Snow Country, Ski, and *Skiing* magazines have tips that hone in on very fine parts of this image. If you're not used to imagery, any moving image you can create of a skier at all is a good first step. As you get better, more and more detail will fill in. Add to this image a feeling of what your muscles are doing and where your own hips, shoulders, legs, feet, and arms are. As your skiing improves so will your image. If you're a visual learner, you'll be able to create much of your image by watching coaches, racers, and instructors on the hill. The best angle to choose is from behind, so try to follow great skiers down the hill, since this is the way your most effective image will be oriented.

Get on Your Marks

The most critical element of Alpine skiing is the correct upright stance from which to spring dynamically into action. Even in pictures of top GS racers blasting their skis around a gate with their legs almost parallel to the slope, their upper body remains upright. The shoulders should remain as level as possible. Hands should be placed out in front of you with a 70-degree angle between your upper and lower arm. The arms should be set several inches to the outside of your body. Since the pole plant is done with a wrist flick, there should be no up-down, front-back, or side-to-side motion of the hands. Knees should be slightly flexed in a basic athletic stance pointed down at the shovel of the ski. The hips should be forward. The upper body should face directly down the hill, unless you are in a long GS traverse. The hips should push forward.

Learn Cues to Guide You

As in all sports, skiing has its own unique cues. Some are very specific: for example, sit on a milk stool as if you were milking a cow. Others are tactical: for example, trace your turn in the snow with your eyes. Still others are feeling cues: for example, feel pressure on the balls of your feet. The following are a sampling of cues that successful coaches use for teaching GS turns.

Pick a line for your turn. Ben Gaylord, Vail's head coach for race clinics, says, "The line is the technique." By picking a nice round C-shaped turn, you have a pretty good chance of good entry into the turn, a nice carve, and a good finish. However, if you pick a Z-shaped turn, you'll use excessive rotation, terrible skidding, and a host of other technical flaws. If you make S turns, you may never learn to finish a turn and will probably skid from one turn to the next.

Picking a line for your turns is a tremendous visual aid. This gives you a wonderful set of cues absent in most other sports. It's like drawing a road you can follow down the slope that avoids ice and rocks. It's a wonderful planning technique. Watch most skiers come down the hill. You'll usually see a very quick turn across the fall line. A C-shaped turn allows you to let your skis go two to three lengths in the fall line, which prevents oversteering and skidding.

Wait for the turn to develop. A rush to get across the fall line quickly causes skis to skid just as a car would if suddenly and radically steered on snow or ice. The combination of a C-shaped turn and allowing your skis to run several lengths in the fall line gives the turn a good chance to develop. If you get going too fast in the fall line, consider a shorter pair of skis with a steeper side cut.

Edge before you steer. This is the single most useful strategy for learning how to carve a turn. Any steering or twisting movement that occurs before a ski is on edge will cause it to skid. Carving after a skid just isn't going to happen. Nearly 100 percent of recreational skiers skid first in a rush to get a turn going into the fall line. To edge first, get your skis to cross under your hips before you start to steer. Take your cue from snowboarders, who move their body over their ski before they start to turn.

Start the turn by shortening the radius. Instead of swiveling or pivoting the ski, start the turn by pressuring the front of the ski once it is on edge. That will steer the turn. Nearly all turns begin with this steering movement.

Control the turn entry to control the turn. Do most of your turning before you hit the fall line. The shape of the hill, gravity, and G forces are all best suited to aid your turning if you do it before the fall line. Look down at recreational skiers from a chairlift and you will see that they grunt, groan, push, and skid most of their turn after the fall line. This is when it is hardest to turn and when turning will do the most to slow you down.

Use the center of the ski to maintain the radius of the turn. This places you in a perfectly centered, stable position.

Use your heels to end the turn. Press directly down through your heel at the end of the turn. Don't press out to the sides of your boots or the ski will skid.

Shift your weight with your feet. Pictures of the French team from the late 1960s show skiers pressuring the backs of their skis, using an exaggerated "sitting-back" position. Modern skis are so sophisticated that it is no longer necessary to move your frame from front to back. With your body balanced over your skis, you can pressure the front of your skis by standing on the balls of your feet, the middle by standing on your arches, and the rear by standing on your heels. Modern turns are so fast that there just isn't the time or the need actually to move your body from front to back during each turn.

Square your shoulders. Shoulders should remain as level as possible without dipping from one side to the other or rotating. Should the shoulders dip on very steep terrain, they should still remain parallel to the hill.

Face downhill. Your head should remain facing down the hill and sit quietly over your upper body.

Ski from a position of maximum strength. The strongest position to resist centrifugal force is with your hip into the hill, your downhill leg nearly straight, your body upright and facing downhill. This places the maximum amount of force on your bones rather than your muscles. There should be a straight line that connects your downhill hip, knee, and ankle. Top racers pressure the skis directly down the length of the ski with their hip, knee, and ankle in that straight line. Pressing the downhill knee into the hill outside this straight line creates lots of excessive pressure on the knee and puts you into a position of weakness.

Move your hips into the hill. The most powerful movement in modern skiing comes from the hips. The hips should move into the hill as much as is necessary to overcome centrifugal force. The best cue is one taught Swiss children: use your belly button as a headlight that always shines down the hill into the valley. To move your hi into this extremely angulated position, try moving your uphill foot forward. The best drill to get a feeling for where the hip should be is to pick up your uphill ski and turn the tip as far downhill as possible as you traverse the slope. Many skiers mistake this hip movement for lowering the hips by flexing the knees. That will cause them to tire very quickly. The downhill leg is actually fairly straight, while the uphill leg is bent as is required by the sharpness of the turn and the steepness of the hill.

Sit on a milk stool. To sink your hips into the hill, pretend your uphill buttock is sitting on a milk stool. With mild angulation, that stool would be on your uphill ski. As you angulate more severely, the stool moves uphill.

Don't come up at the end of the turn. The old school would have a skier come up at the end of the turn to unweight the skis. While that can still help in really bad crud or windblown powder, it's no longer necessary on groomed terrain. Skis are so light and spring off the snow so easily, you just don't need to unweight the skis. Mike Porter, director of the Vail/Beaver Creek Ski School, points out that the energy from the end of the turn is completely wasted if you use it to stand up. Rather you should use that energy to get your skis under your hips and into the next turn.

Move your hips forward and across your skis at the beginning of the turn. Many coaches believe that the hips are used to initiate the new turn since they represent the center of mass that you want to move. The hips are much more powerful than the knees. A good cue is to move them up and across your skis at an angle 45 degrees from the tip. I like the feeling of getting the hips to accelerate forward across the fall line and then facing directly downhill during the carving part of the turn.

Feel with your feet. The feet have always been great cues for Alpine skiers. For decades coaches have asked racers to "feel" the snow. During the first edge set, the ankle strikes the front inside of the boot. The ball of the foot is firmly pressed upon. The middle of the turn is executed with pressure on the arch of the foot. Extreme pressure can be put on the heel, but you shouldn't press any farther back onto the rear of your boot. If you feel that, you're too far back.

Bend your knees into your ski tips. Knee angulations are popular in short slalom turns when the skier stands on the balls of his feet, jams the edges, and steers the skis. For GS turns, the knees should drive down into the ski tips without angulating much into the turn.

Use your poles as a viewing box. Hold the poles in front of you as a gate through which to watch what is in front of you. This should keep your upper body and hips facing squarely down the hill.

Feel your lats. To get the feeling of the severely angulated turns you see on the World Cup circuit, as your hip goes further into the hill, you should feel tremendous pressure on your lats. These large back muscles hold the upper body upright.

Get Good Error Correction

As part of researching this chapter I spent three days with Ben Gaylord, head coach of race clinics at Vail. They were among the best motor-learning experiences I've had. Ben would say, "OK, keep your shoulders level." He'd imitate my error so I could see it, then show me the correct technique, then show me a drill to make it sink in. In this way he could fix one problem after another with the workmanlike precision of a surgeon. Here are some examples of common errors.

Swiveling the foot to begin the turn. Many skiers step onto the uphill ski and swivel it underfoot before edging the ski, which results in a skidded turn. Any attempt to carve after pivoting the ski will result in more skidding. By moving the hip up and across the ski, setting an edge, and then steering, this error is corrected.

Rotating the upper body to initiate a turn. Many skiers unconsciously rotate their shoulders, hands, and arms to initiate a turn. Practice skiing holding both poles horizontal to the snow in front of you. Keep your shoulders and your hands pointing straight down the hill as you turn. That will keep your upper body from initiating the turn and force you to initiate your turn with your lower body.

Using a Z turn. Look at most recreational skiers on a moderately steep slope and you will see them make Z turns. To get across the fall line as quickly as possible, they will severely skid the ski across the hill into a traverse. The actual shape of the turn is a Z as in Zorro. There is no possibility of carving a Z turn. By allowing the ski to stay in the fall line for two or three lengths, there is a much better chance of making a carved C turn. This is how the line you choose determines the technique you will use.

Letting the arms stray. Skiing provides the opportunity for as many extraneous movements as tennis. In skiing, most are in the upper body. Arms go up and down, back and forth. The shoulders dip left and right. You may protest "not me" and maybe you're right, but first look at a video. Skiing with your poles held horizontally in front of you is the best way to see what happens. If you watch your poles, you'll see them drop if you drop a shoulder. You'll also see them rotate if that's how you initiate your turns.

Tune in to Onboard Feedback

I learned that I truly can't ski and chew gum at the same time. While I'd monitor my shoulders, my hips would go in the wrong direction. Once I got my hips set, I'd push my hands the wrong way. But bit by bit, each component became more automatic. That's why a body scan works so well, focusing on one area of the body, then moving to another. For instance, you might feel the pressure on the soles of your feet moving from the balls of your feet to the arches to the heels during a turn, and then concentrate on feeling the inside front part of your boot as you initiate a turn.

Remember that the feet are giving you feedback on what has already taken place. Mike Porter, director of the Vail/Beaver Creek Ski School, says, "If you're looking for foot feel, you're feeling for history." Mike also believes that if you tune into too many "feelings" when you ski, you will suffer from sensory overload, becoming overwhelmed with the data.

Since you can look out and see your hands, you've got great visual feedback to be certain they are where they are supposed to be. Visual feedback will also tell you whether you have carved the shape of the turn you want. You can also look back in the snow to see which part of your turn is skidded and which is carved. I also like to scan different body parts at different stages of the turn. I'll monitor the ball of my foot during turn initiation as I'm watching the part of the turn I want. Then I may check my hands to make certain they stay still during the pole plant. You can develop your own scan. Only a coach, an instructor, or a video camera can confirm what you feel. If they do, hold on to that feeling because you can use it to perform that part of the turn correctly from then on. In fact "getting it" often means finding the right feel. You can also monitor for mistakes. If your thighs are screaming, check to see if you're not excessively bent back over the ends of your skis. Look to see if your hand is coming around in back of you.

Play It Back

I practice skiing year-round through mental imagery. The better the image, the better you'll ski, even if it's just for one week a year. I try to picture myself from the front and back. I also try to feel my shoulders, thighs, feet, and other body parts so that I have a real living image of skiing. As you read articles or see races on TV, you can incorporate new bits and pieces into your image. If it doesn't fit, you may make a breakthrough by figuring out how to fit a new maneuver into your image. Most important, anytime you learn something new, add it to your image that evening and play it back until it's hard-wired. Good skiers come back for the next season better than at the end of the last because they have further enhanced their image over the summer.

Learn How You Learn

As you try some of the sample tips above, see which ones work best. If they don't make much sense, but you try them over and over and suddenly "get it," you're learning by doing. If you like the more mechanical cues because they make sense to you, you may learn by analysis. If you learn best by looking at race footage, pictures, and good skiers and coaches, you're a visual learner. If you learn by feeling, you'll rely heavily on feeling with your feet. Remember that dominant learning styles are very important at the beginning. As you improve, remember to go back to other learning styles to further enhance your progress. Although you may have a dominant learning style, try to use every channel you can for learning. The cues above reflect a wide range of different ways of learning. Skiing is the first sport where learning styles have been widely applied. Now most ski schools are aware of different learning styles. Once you know how you learn best, try to find that kind of teaching.

Skiing is almost unique among sports in that breakthroughs come in surprising and unexpected ways, which is why it's important to tune into a variety of ways of learning.

Remove Physical Impediments

There are lots of muscles that can be skied into shape. The biggest exception is the thigh. At the Vail race program last year, all of the injuries were among those athletes who did not do adequate dry-land training. Unless your quads are strong enough to handle the forces of skiing and have a full range of motion, you'll be severely limited. High-level skiing takes enormous strength and explosiveness. Without the proper strength training, it's very hard to improve. The vast majority of recreational skiers simply do not have the strength to ski medium-speed carved turns, deep powder, or a long line of steep bumps. Strong quads are also the best protection against knee injuries. Alberto Tomba's thighs give him a big reserve of strength. Tomba was born with most of his strength. Mere mortals have to build that with squats. Squat strength can be transferred better to the hill than any other form of weight training. However, squat strength alone won't increase the instantaneous power that gold medalists have. What will? High-speed exercises that rely only on body weight called plyometrics. Lunges are one highly effective plyometric for skiing used by Tomba.

Most adults can't afford to ski all week and so can't really ski themselves into shape. You can get your endurance strength from rollerblades and stairclimbers. Both offer you excellent conditioning during the week and can put you in great shape on the snow. Blading is so close to downhill skiing that U.S. Olympic Team members are actually taught technique on rollerblades. In New York, I practice Nordic skating technique on the uphills and Alpine slalom or GS technique on the downhills. Friend after friend over forty makes the same claim: blading gets them into super shape for skiing. If you have only one way to condition for skiing, this is it.

Road cycling conditions the thighs for endurance, but it won't give you the power nor will it give you the holding strength for riding a flat thigh down the mountain. However, mountain biking over rough terrain on a single track develops the thigh strength and uncannily similar steering and body angulation movements you need in skiing.

Look at a photo of a racer rounding the end of a turn through a GS gate. You'll notice tremendous projection of the ski away from the body. That's possible only with greatly improved hip flexibility. Most adults' hips are so tight that they are almost locked in chains. Chapter 26, "Building Elastic Muscle," has terrific exercises to open up your hips.

Find the Right Coach

More and more men are entering race programs to learn how to ski better. Even if you have no racing aspirations, consider a race program for making big breakthroughs in your skiing. At the end of a day's racing clinic, you can see improvements on the second hand. That gives you positive feedback that you really are better. Error corrections tend to be very focused in race programs. Coaches are so used to looking for and fixing technical faults that you're apt to achieve fast results.

Chapter 18

Aerobic Tennis

THE SUN SANK INTO THE OCEAN, SPRINKLING A PALETTE OF PASTELS ONTO the green and pink tennis bungalows at the La Costa Resort and Spa in Carlsbad, California. On court nine, my lungs were burning, my eyes hurt, and my back was killing me. From forehand to backhand, volley to overhead, back to front, I was getting killed on every shot. My opponent? A seventy-three-year-old man named Pancho Segura. I undertook a tennis odyssey for this book to find the best tennis pros in the country. Everyone said Pancho was the best. Pancho arrived at the fountain of youth before me and drank it dry.

> Conventional Wisdom:
> > *Tennis is a semi-sedentary gentleman's game that is declining in popularity.*
>
> New Paradigm:
> > *You haven't seen Agassi play.*

Tennis is the intersection of everything I've learned writing this book and is the best sport in which to see the profound impact nutrition, talent advancement, technology, flexibility, and weight training can have. Tennis will help you accumulate speed, agility, power, endurance, and skill. I've titled this chapter "Aerobic Tennis" because the sport delivers a terrific aerobic workout that rivals running or cycling. During the dark cold days of winter or on the road, when it's hard to motivate yourself to work out, an hour on the court with a good teaching pro or disciplined partner delivers the goods.

WHY YOU SHOULD PLAY TENNIS

Learn to Learn

The best evidence that men can learn sports extremely well as adults is appearing on the senior men's tennis circuit. Men who never picked up the game until adulthood are now playing competitively against the Wimbledon players of twenty years ago. How? They bring lots of power, strength, and fitness from general conditioning, an aggressive attitude, and well-honed stroke mechanics. There's even an eighty-five-and-over singles division. Vic Braden says, "They're animals!"

Tennis has another big bonus. Although tennis is a complex sport of multi-limb coordination, you can learn how to gain lots of talent without getting hurt. If you're learning how to learn in windsurfing or skiing, mistakes can launch you off the head of the board or into the woods.

Increase Aerobic Power

The average play in tennis is so short that even the pros don't get much of an aerobic workout during competition. Top draws can play a three-hour Wimbledon match and be in motion for less than half an hour. However, you can get a great aerobic workout with extensive side-to-side and backcourt-to-net drills if a friend or coach is willing to feed you balls. With a heart-rate monitor to keep score, my heart rate stays over 130 for an entire hour with long bursts at 150 beats a minute. That gives me tremendous skill training and an aerobic workout to boot — pure play with a great payoff.

Develop Power

True power in any sport requires the successful linking of each body part. Mastering the proper force production of legs, hips, shoulders,

233

upper arm, forearm, and wrist can be transferred to any sport requiring power generated from the legs up. Even the slightest of players can generate enormous force by linking these elements.

Goal Setting for Those Tough Days in the Gym

Tennis provides wonderful feedback for all the effort put in at the gym. Whatever goals you choose begin to pay off by the first weekend's play. More powerful thighs explode you toward the ball faster, stronger forearms dampen the impact of the ball, a stronger back and chest give you more oomph with each stroke.

Develop Footwork

Watch Stefan Edberg play the net. He has tremendous grace and presence that would be an asset in any sport. If you've ever felt uncoordinated, this is the opportunity to develop the balletlike grace of a top player.

Develop Hand-Eye Coordination

Andre Agassi's game is built off phenomenal hand speed, coordination, and accuracy. A western forehand will develop great tennis hands.

Portability

Tennis is as portable a fitness sport as running. If you develop an aerobic game, you can get the equivalent of an hour's run in an hour's tennis. If you travel, it's easier to find a court and a pro for an hour of aerobic tennis drills than it is to find a new jogging, blading, or cycling course.

Develop Quickness

Where running is sure to slow most people down, tennis can make you really quick. Tennis is all about explosive speed. If you can explode with your first step toward the ball and settle in to hit, your accuracy will skyrocket. Unfortunately, many players move slowly off the mark and are still settling in when they hit the ball so they are off balance.

Acquire Grace

Properly learned, tennis will give you the grace and elegance that will help the way you move in any sport. Tennis allows you to develop and keep a basic athletic stance under pressure.

SPORTS-IMPROVEMENT TECHNOLOGY

Years ago you couldn't play pro tennis if you couldn't hit the ball near dead center of the racquet. Now many more men can play high-level tennis because the new technology gives them 37 percent more power with off-center hits. That means less-than-perfect hand-eye coordination can still deliver shots that are winners. If this technology had been perfected during the height of the tennis craze, many more men would have stayed in the game, because they would have attained a much higher level of play. Tennis, like skiing, is a sport where the technique is the technology. That is, the technology coaxes you to play in a certain way. The wrong technology encourages you to develop short, choppy strokes and a game that is high on power and low on precision.

Dr. Carl Hedrik, a professor of mechanical engineering at the University of California, Berkeley, believes that there are three important characteristics of the present-day tennis racquet that enhance performance. These features have evolved over the last twenty-five years.

Traditional tennis racquets were made of wood, which is an extremely flexible material. "If you try to make it stiff, it gets very big and heavy and it has a lot of damping in it so you lose a lot of energy. The energy that the human puts into the ball is lost in the racquet," says Dr. Hedrik.

In the early 1960s the first nonwood racquet, known as the T2000, was introduced by La Coste. "This stainless steel racquet with the tiny little head that Connors used forever really started the materials revolution," says Dr. Hedrik.

After the T2000, designers tried an aluminum racquet, then a racquet of aluminum on the outside with a composite material on the inside. Designers at that point became interested in the strength-to-weight ratio. Dr. Hedrik says, "These new materials were allowing the racquets to be stronger and lighter, so the strength-to-weight ratio was going way, way up. In the old days, to make it stronger, it had to be heavier. Now you could make a racquet that was both stronger and lighter. Today a graphite composite is used. It's the best because it allows the racquet to be stiff and light at the same time.

"The sweet spot on a conventional racquet," says Dr. Hedrik, "was way down in the throat someplace, and no one was ever hitting it." The oversize head brought the center of percussion down to the geometric center of the racquet. The sweet spot on the racquet today coincides with the center of the strung area. Now, when you try to hit the ball in the center of the racquet, you are also trying to hit it at the center of percussion. It is the sweet spot." This in combination with the material composites allowed for larger racquet faces and lighter racquets. It gave the designers a tremendous amount of freedom.

"Wide body" refers to the thickness of the racquet. "A wide-bodied racquet allows the racquet to be very, very stiff, so virtually no energy is lost when you hit the ball. You become a more precise player because the racquet no longer bends and flexes in funny ways. Also, because the racquet doesn't bend, energy isn't lost in the flexibility of the racquet. Because the racquet is hollow inside, it's full of air, so it's very, very good for vibration absorption," says Dr. Hedrik.

All three of these characteristics aid in player performance. Dr. Hedrik adds that players today can get away with a shorter swing. "You don't have to hit as hard to get the ball back deep. Another way this has helped performance is that it's during the big, long swing where all the error in the wrists and strokes occurs. When players swing shorter, there's less margin for error."

Stuart Chirls, associate editor of *Tennis* magazine, says, "The wide-body racquet allows you to hit many times harder than you would with a narrow racquet, with the same effort. It's amazing. It's the difference between an aluminum and a wooden bat in baseball."

Last summer my father was seventy-eight years old. He was getting beaten by many of his friends at the game he loves best, tennis. I suggested that what he needed was a new racquet. He had resisted for nearly a decade succumbing to wide bodies because he saw his friends develop crippling tennis elbows and an unenviable loss of control. Each one of them had bought an early wide body. They developed very short, punchlike poaching shots, but their ground strokes went flying. I encouraged my father to get a skill-improvement racquet, which gave him some power but lots of control. The first time he played with it I was stunned when he returned a heavy, deep-to-his-backhand topspin with a nice solid thwack down the baseline. His net game went from a nice poaching game to a solid, offensive put-away. He played a good fifteen years younger by playing up to the racquet.

What to Look for in Today's Racquets

Lighter weight. Lighter weights mean greater maneuverability. You'll be able to get the racquet around much faster.

Less vibration. Less vibration means you can hit harder without losing control, risking injury, or suffering through play with hard-hitting players.

Denser stringing. Theory says that the more strings you get on a ball the better the control. New racquets now come with much denser stringing patterns. Head's Andre Agassi racquet is one example.

Bigger sweet spot. This is where it all began for tennis. Now racquets advertise "the biggest sweet spot of all." As you get older, a bigger sweet spot becomes critical. If you miss a step or get to the ball late, you're more likely to hit off-center.

Greater flexibility. A very stiff wide-body racquet almost stops your stroke at impact. The more flexible, highly damped racquets allow you to accelerate through a hard ball for lots of drive. These racquets encourage great stroke mechanics and the full use of your body to hit the ball. If nothing else, they make tennis a much more athletic game.

Curiously, almost none of the pros use thick, wide-body racquets.

They'd prefer to generate the force themselves or take it off their opponent's ball. But even the pros take advantage of the increased racquet power by taking much shorter backswings. The length on their stroke comes in the follow-through. Vic Braden says, "Most pros don't want to change because their motor program 'software package' is highly tuned and new racquets scare the heck out of them."

GETTING GOOD FAST

Create an Image

The most effective new means of creating a proper image is with a photomontage. This gives you a series of still pictures to study the motion that a top pro uses. More clearly than with videotape or personal instruction, you can see where each body segment is throughout the strike. Many of the popular tennis magazines now employ this technique. Sybervision has a repetitive sequence of shots that can help you start to paint an image. Unfortunately, the tapes I reviewed were of fairly old technique. You can create your own tapes by taping matches on ESPN, ESPN2, CBS, USA, or other television stations. On cable there is nearly always a tennis match playing. Replay it in slow motion on your VCR. Try to scan a picture for a particular body part. For instance, look to see how far back the racquet comes on the forehand. Then look for foot position. In this way you can construct a first-rate image. Ask your instructor or good players you know to show you a motion in real time and slow motion. Watching matches in person gives you an added third dimension. Try to watch one feature at a time.

Get on Your Marks

The easiest and best way to get good fast is to get your body into the most efficient biomechanical position before you set your body into motion. You vastly reduce the number of variables that can go wrong. You can practice getting on your marks in your office, bedroom, or even as you fall asleep, so that you have a rock-solid preparatory position.

I love the Agassi/Courier style of game just because it demands and builds so much more athleticism. You push with your legs, lunge with your body, thrust with your hips. It's just a terrific workout and looks spectacular. I like it, too, because you can whack the ball as hard as you want and it will still go in because of the awesome top-spin. This chapter reflects that prejudice and the hope that you will try a new motor-learning experience by trying the new game.

Right-handed Western Forehand
- Left foot points at your opponent.
- Right foot points at the sideline.
- Left shoulder is tucked under your chin.
- Elbow is raised and points to the rear fence. Pros go even further and bring the elbow around to 200 degrees from the net.
- Right hand faces the ground.
- Racquet is in within your eyesight and no more than 55 degrees back in relation to net. There's much more power to be unleashed by cocking the body than there is by a little bit more arm extension. Courier uses only about a 55 to 65 degree backswing, which is tiny compared to the 90 to 180 degrees most players take. This short backswing forces you to use your body to get a much longer follow-through.
- Hips point at least toward the sideline, farther back if possible. I like to call this the trigger position where every muscle, tendon, and joint is ready to be applied with maximum force. You can actually look at each body part to make certain that it's where you think it is.

Learn Cues to Guide You

Cues go from very simple, biomechanically sound, easily remembered hints to the very complex. For instance, if you are going to learn the monster flail — that is, opening your body up before you hit — then you need to be able to execute properly the complete opening-up sequence from shoulder roll through hip thrust. You need a highly developed sense of where all these body parts are and how they work together before you can consider executing it. If you are one of the few truly right-brained athletes who can pick that sequence up just by looking, you can stop reading here. Most of us need several very simple cues we can lock on to to help us guide the racquet where we want it. Some players like to focus on just a single cue. Most can't handle more than three at a time. Here are sample cues for the forehand.

Keep your palm going toward your opponent. Tom Salmon from the Topnotch at Stowe Resort and Spa in Stowe, Vermont, says the hand is the best and simplest cue to use. Let the hand go to the ball and through the ball toward the target as fast and accurately as possible and as far forward as your body extension will allow. Use every last body segment to reach as far forward with your hand as you can. Think about letting your hand follow straight toward the target longer.

Catch your stroke arm. This is a terrific cue because it gives your strokes an endpoint. If you have a good on-your-marks position, catching your arm at the end gives you a perfect stopping point to groove your forehand with. This prevents you from over-rotating.

Open up. In major ball sports, including golf and baseball, players begin their swing with the body. That generates more power. In tennis, opening the body first allows you to start momentum moving at the ball without making a final commitment to where your racquet must go. To do this, bring your shoulder forward, then your hip, and finally your arm. It can also pre-stretch the muscles for even more power.

Let the racquet come below the ball. Vic Braden talks about pointing at the ball with the left hand, then letting the right hand fall 30 degrees below it. The body comes down with the arm and then back up. The arm follows through to a point 45 degrees above the horizontal. Most players get stuck right at the horizontal. This forces them to generate topspin. Touring pros say they get all their topspin through rotational forces in the shoulder, arm, and hand, so they can hit through flat but still develop a lot of spin. While that's true, it takes a very advanced player to execute a Western-grip topspin with a flat stroke.

Accelerate. Make no mistake about it, the way to better tennis and less injury is increasing the velocity at which you strike the ball with mechanically perfect form. Many men try to hit a hard ball by muscling it, which leads to overuse injuries. That's why strength alone can be dangerous. A much better solution is to add rapid acceleration throughout the shot with a flexible racquet. Since timing is so critical to acceleration, get moving forward into the ball, then line up your footwork, then get your body moving, then your arm, then accelerate. Curiously, just the sensation of acceleration itself is a great cue. Your hand is the most sensitive part of your upper arm to acceleration and is your best cue.

Keep your shoulders level. Dipping your shoulders will launch a ball over the fence. Go down for a ball with your knees, not your shoulders or back.

Hit with your shoulder. The shoulder is the cannon of good ground strokes. By cocking your shoulders at least 100 degrees away from the net, you cork up the largest amount of potential force with which to hit the ball.

Stop your body to get more power. Open up your hips until your belly button faces the net. Stop your body there and let your hand and arm whip through the end of the shot. That accelerates the ball 1.5 times faster than letting your body continue through the shot, according to measurements made by coach Vic Braden.

Keep your elbow close for power. Keep your elbow close to your body. The farther it is from your body, the less power you have. Vic Braden says that it should be no more than eight inches away.

Watch the ball. As obvious as this sounds, photographs of most players who mishit the ball show them looking up and away from the ball.

Begin by imagining where the ball is going to go based on the way your opponent is set up to hit it, then track it from your opponent's racquet. The best tip is to look at the ball for the direction of spin. That will force you to really sharpen your focus so you actually see it after the bounce and can plan for topspin, underspin, or sidespin. Although you can't see the ball hit your racquet, photos of the top players show their eyes tightly focused on the point of impact. Most amateurs don't follow the ball into the racquet, because it takes too much concentration and too much effort to refocus from far vision to near vision. They may also make the mistake of looking at their opponent before the shot is finished.

Turn first, then run. If you run sideways, your eyes go up and down too much to be able to follow the ball accurately. Start with long steps, then shorten them as you approach the hitting zone so that you can precisely adjust your stance before you hit. Spend the last second before you hit the ball adjusting your stance, not scrambling into position.

Get balanced and in position before you hit. Hitting off-balance trashes accuracy and power.

Explode toward the ball. The most important move in tennis is the exploding first step toward the ball. That gives you your only real chance to get to the ball and get stabilized well enough to hit from a position of strength and balance. Lots of men have great ground strokes, but they don't amount to much once they're on the move.

Practice the Four Rs. Butch Young of Vic Braden's Tennis College reminded me of these:

> Ready position.
> Read the ball.
> React to the ball's spin.
> Recover quickly.

Get Good Error Correction

Even if you don't have a great eye for the way other people play, you can develop a very good eye for how *you* play. For ground strokes position a video camera on a table next to the net facing your service line. The newer cameras with built-in viewing screens are ideal for on-court feedback. Here are easy errors to look for.

Don't lift your head. With accelerating ground strokes, there is a tendency to tighten the neck and shoulder muscles, thereby lifting the head with the shot. The cue is to practice a totally relaxed neck and shoulder musculature to leave the head as a completely independent unit. In that way you can keep your head down like a golfer.

Don't muscle the ball. If your shoulder and elbow hurt and you notice grinding noises in your shoulder and back, you may be muscling the ball. Tom Salmon, the director of the highly rated Tennis Center at the Topnotch at Stowe Resort and Spa in Stowe, Vermont, recommends accelerating more through the ball to prevent the low-speed push through the ball known as muscling. Acceleration gives the very pleasant sensation of power and muscle relaxation.

Don't over-rotate the shoulder. This pulls you past the point of getting any power. Better to stop when your belly button faces the net.

Don't bend at the waist. This puts tremendous strain on your lower back. As you rise to hit the ball, you're likely to whip your head up with your body. A better solution is to lower your body with your legs.

Don't get your arm stuck behind you. Out of sight, out of mind is what happens with arm awareness. If your backswing goes past the point you can see it, it's too far back.

Don't tip the shoulders. Keep them square and level rather than see-sawing them up and down.

Don't get your center of gravity caught back. You'll discover this if you're always hitting off your back foot. That means that none of your mass or power is going forward into the ball.

Don't come up in the middle of the shot. There's a big tendency with topspin forehands to come up very abruptly low-to-high and end the shot way short. The pros actually hit a pretty flat shot and let the natural rotation of the arm create the topspin. Better to come through the ball, then use your forearm and/or wrist at the end of the stroke aggressively.

Tune in to Onboard Feedback

Visual. Well-trained eyes find the likely path of your opponent's shots, the spin of the ball, and the result of your impact on the ball. I use my peripheral vision to see the path the racquet traveled through during the last part of the stroke to make certain it went forward and not down on the volley. You can also see the conclusion of your ground strokes to make certain that your forearm came through and then up toward your opposite ear and shoulder.

Power sense. Get a feel for accelerating racquet speed.

Position sense. In the setup, sense where your elbow, shoulders, hips, and feet are.

Use a Checklist

Checklists give you a way to work on your game every time you play. Pick two or three items to concentrate on, then rotate new items in. Upgrade your checklist as your game improves.

Remove Physical Impediments

Strong, explosive thigh muscles make the biggest single difference in good tennis. They allow you to lower your body to the ball and spring forward into each shot. Tennis is called a game of fast feet and slow hands. Getting to the ball quickly means an explosive first step. Without strong, explosive thigh muscles, you'll overwork your back bending down to balls or rotate too much instead of hitting through the ball. The keys to explosiveness are strong, powerful quads. Squats prepare the base. With really strong quads, you can sink and wait for a ball and then rise through it and hit it. Without strong quads pushing you up into the ball, you'll lose loads of power.

The greatest fear of many players is a torn Achilles tendon. All any orthopedic surgeon will tell you about preventing one is to keep stretching it. For this reason, active strengthening stretching exer-

Sample Forehand Checklist
- Explode to the ball.
- Take short steps on the final approach.
- Open up on your upper body before coming through with your hand.
- Aim at the inside of the ball as it approaches your racquet.
- Bring the elbow straight through close to the body.
- Push your hand at and through the ball.
- Focus on acceleration.
- Stop your body when your belly button faces the net.
- Don't step through with your back foot but allow it to be pulled through.
- End up with hand between shoulder and ear.

cises, described in Chapter 26, "Building Elastic Muscle," are crucial to remaining injury free.

Upper-body strength development allows you to hit through the ball with more punch. Wrist extensors and flexors, biceps, triceps, and pecs all help you hit through the ball with more strength. Deltoid lifts protect the shoulder and improve strength for the serve. Research at Pennsylvania State University demonstrates that strength training can increase the power of your shots by 35 percent.

Faster reaction time can be built by playing more doubles, playing on very fast courts, especially at altitude, or playing squash. Squash players have the best net reaction time in the game. Curiously, many players believe that one game ruins shots for the other. Motor-learning experts say that's just not true.

Think Biomechanics

The final force that drives a tennis ball from the ground strokes to the serve comes from the ground up. The force begins with foot drive, moves to the quads, pushes through the hips, and ends with the arm. Any time you hit, feel where the power comes from. The reason kids hit so hard is that they have excellent biomechanics, linking one part of the body to the other from the ground up. The final result is the speed you can get the racquet head to when it hits the ball.

Find the Right Coach

More than any other sport, tennis has huge variability in teaching styles and methods. But there's a big problem that goes beyond that — content. I had four nationally respected, even famous, coaches show me four completely different and contradictory forehands. Even within a single program, there are radical differences in what pupils are taught. At La Costa on a Saturday afternoon, Pancho Segura told me I should stick with the continental grip for the service, as most good coaches suggest. One hour later, another instructor had me roll over toward a Western grip, exactly what Pancho warned me not to do. The other coach says he gets more people to play like this, then confides that this is what he teaches women who don't play very much. In a twelve-hour period instructors suggested four different elbow positions for my forehand. Where lies the truth? Finally Pancho introduced me to a touring pro named Martin. Like athletes at the top end of their game, he was "consciously competent" with a great understanding of exactly what to do and how to show it to me. He told me I was losing power because I didn't cock my hips as well as my shoulders. I did this. Pow! The ball clocked the net at Mach 2! I resolved to meet up with Martin and start learning from the playing pros. Judge for yourself who makes sense, then build your own game. I'm thoroughly convinced that too many coaches are just plain bluffing. Be tough! Make the coach make you get each point.

So many body parts move so quickly in a fraction of a second that it usually requires an analysis of high-speed video to dissect your form. A coach with a great eye can do that dissection, imitate your errors, and demonstrate the correct technique. Where many ski instructors can readily mimic errors and explain error correction, I've found that few tennis instructors have that capability. They'll show you what to do, but can't adequately show you what you're doing wrong.

Tennis instructors have much more of an attitude problem than almost all instructors except ski teachers. They display their perfect smooth stroke and fire off a torrent of commands that are hard to comprehend and impossible to follow. It's the rare teacher who has the eye, the understanding, and the patience to help you make big gains. It shouldn't be that way.

Tennis is a sport where the level of play is very precisely graded. When you work on a shot, say a two-handed backhand, you should be able to achieve a good down-the-line and cross-court shot to within two feet of the baseline on a consistent basis. You should see those shots improve with each lesson. If you're not getting these results, find another coach.

Chapter 19

Power Blading

THE GULF WAR WAS ONLY TWO DAYS OLD AND MY SHINS WERE KILLING me. I had arrived in Dhahran, Saudi Arabia, with a pair of sneakers and no other exercise gear, expecting that the ground war would start shortly and we'd be stationed somewhere up near the front on the Kuwaiti border. When we learned there would be a prolonged air war, I took to running daily, which I hadn't done for years. There are no hills in the Eastern Province of Saudi Arabia, so all my road-work was confined to a hard cement sidewalk along the water's edge. In desperation I called my wife and asked her to have my new roll-erblades shipped to me. By the end of the week, relief for my aching shins had arrived in the form of a five-wheeled pair of Racerblades.

Early the following morning I prepared for my first skate in the hotel parking lot. The town cleared out after the first Scud attacks, so the roads by the hotel were pretty empty. I got down into my best imitation Eric Heiden low tuck with one hand on my back, the other slowly moving alongside my body, and my legs pushing evenly out to the side. I had earphones under my civil defense helmet with my Walkman playing "Ba Ba Ba Ba Barbara Ann," nerve gas injectors on my left hip, and a gas mask on my right. That first day I heard the air raid sirens wail just as I came up on a great white mosque. Fortunately, I had on elbow and knee protectors so I could slide into a building across from the mosque. I heard several locals look at me in scorn, saying, "Who is the infidel?" The Scud missed.

Conventional Wisdom:
Blading is for kids.
New Paradigm:
Blading will make you a kid again.

I returned to Vermont at the end of the Gulf War for a weekend's skiing. I was prepared to be in terrible ski shape. To my delight, the rollerblades had provided such terrific cross training that I jumped onto my skis like I'd never been off. But the biggest and most pleasant surprise was that my knees, which had been pretty painful the previous year, seemed like new. During two months in Saudi Arabia, I'd started skating with my legs nearly straight. As I got better, I slowly sank into a lower position by bending my legs about 5 percent more each week. In retrospect, my gradually improving knees followed classical physical therapy theory: extend the range of motion by several degrees at a time, gradually building up to a complete range of motion. Blading sure did the trick by rehabilitating my knees better than any conventional surgical technique. I was sold on blading. Outside of the occasional collision with the pavement, this sport is incredibly easy on the body, great cross training, and fun.

Blading is the best modern sport for athlete building. That's my personal belief. Lots of other sports require certain talents that you must build first in order to enjoy the sport. But the more you blade, with proper knowledge of technique, the more talent you build.

WHY YOU SHOULD BLADE

Power

Blading builds fantastic dynamic power in the muscles of the thighs, hamstrings, and buttocks. These muscles are required in tennis, squash, Alpine skiing, cross-country skiing, cycling, waterskiing, snowboarding, and a range of other sports from basketball to hockey.

As you learn to lower your hips more and more into your stride, you create wonderful dynamic power. I call it dynamic because it gives you speed, power, and explosiveness in one sport after another. You'll be amazed how much faster you sprint to the net in tennis or power through a carved turn in skiing.

Knees

Blading builds great knees. At least 60 percent of the knee's strength is based on the strength of your thigh muscles. The slowly progressive nature of training sinks your body into a position that trains more and more muscle each week. This gradually builds very strong knees that stay strong in ball sports, skiing, and cycling. I really like blading for chondromalacia, an annoying condition where the normally porcelain-smooth undersurface of the kneecap becomes rough and causes a sharp pain when the knee is bent.

Skill

I can't think of another sport that builds so much skill so quickly. You learn terrific balance. You have an opportunity to build a very sophisticated motor program in an easy, effective, piece-by-piece manner. Every day I learn something new about skating. One day I may learn how to get my hips farther into a turn. On another it may be correct arm position. Most important, you learn a dynamic athletic stance, one from which you can aggressively lunge into action.

Heart and Lungs

I unquestionably get my best urban workout on skates. My heart rate is a good thirty beats a minute higher than in any other aerobic activity. As you get into your forties, you look with delight at the heart-rate monitor when it cranks up into the red zone, because it's so hard to get it there otherwise. Some of this increased rate may be caused by the tension in the quadriceps necessary to maintain the correct position, but a lot of it still comes from good hard work. What runners will quickly appreciate is that spreading the load of exercise over bigger muscle groups takes away the pain and yet gives the heart a much hardier workout. While running stresses the small muscles of the calves, blading adds the quads, hamstrings, and buttock muscles.

Back

Blading will kill or cure your back. If you overdo it, your back will feel like it's on fire. This is not a surgical emergency. It's just overuse of vastly underused small back muscles. If you build your back up to tolerate even half an hour of skating on a regular basis, you will have one strong back that's just never going to give out. Remember that the muscles that line the spinal column down the center of your back are quite small and are tightly wrapped, so that swelling can really hurt.

Safety

Because of the wheel-based nature of the sport, the margin of error is huge compared to ice. Your wheels aren't going to slide out from under you easily. You won't go skidding across the ice Dan Jansen–style into the bleachers. Most skaters increase their aggressiveness in line with their level of skill. If you wear the proper safety equipment, you run less of a risk of real injury than when cycling, running, or aerobic dancing. Unless you hit the ground with your body, blading is the ultimate nonimpact sport. It's very easy and even kind to your knees and hips. I've fallen at 30 mph with protective gear and skated away with just a minor scrape.

Doctors are concerned about the risk of injury from explosive movement in the more injury-prone older athlete. Without the pounding of running or potential muscle tearing of sprinting, your risk of injury is very small.

Skate to Ski

Skating is superb cross training for Alpine skiing. Top ski academies now teach their students Alpine technique on rollerblades. By using a consistent surface and pitch (which is very hard to find on snow) many skiers improve dramatically on skates.

Portability

Skating equipment is really easy to take along on a trip. I call a local skating store ahead of time to make certain there is a convenient bike or skate path.

Great Crossover to Speed Skating on Ice

KC Boutiette, an amateur blade racer, made his way to the U.S. Olympic trials. Once there, he borrowed ice blades to exchange for the wheels on his boots. His first time ever on ice, he made the U.S. Olympic team going to Lillehammer. Nice going, KC! The Speedskating Federation now views rollerblading as a tremendous way to grow the size of its talent pool.

SPORTS-IMPROVEMENT TECHNOLOGY

Blading technology improves almost weekly. That's good news, because a bigger wallet for better technology will put you way out in front of the kids. Here's what really works:

Light High-tech Boots

If you want to go fast, you need fast boots. The best boot technology comes from ice speed skating, which is the fastest self-propelled sport in the world, with speeds approximating 40 mph. My first serious boots were Bonts. They're made by an Australian company, are low-cut, and have a hard-molded fiberglass lower and a form-fitting top that can be molded to your foot.

But some very good skaters consider the Bonts too restrictive. If you want less support, you can buy Riedell, Viking, or Interapps boots. However, you'll need lots of experience and really strong ankles for those. The Bonts can accommodate a relative novice with lots of support. If you're one of those people who have always wobbled on ice, you needn't fear blades. You can move the rollers from one side of the boot to the other so that you're perfectly aligned on top of them and needn't worry about your foot caving in to one side or the other. With the right boot, you can ideally position the ball of your foot directly over your wheels.

I bought my first pair of racing boots from Marty Hill at Built for Speed in Syracuse, New York. He said, "You really want these boots to be tight." I didn't quite take him seriously because I had heard the horror stories about painful boots. Marty was right. After boots are broken in, there will be increased slop. My recommendation is that you get boots with these characteristics:

- Your toes should touch the end of the boot without being scrunched.
- The boot should fit around your heel snugly. Once you have tightly buckled your boot you shouldn't be able to move your heel, even if you stand on your toes.
- Your instep should be solidly planted against the sole of the boot.
- Your foot shouldn't collapse into your instep.
- There should be no focal painful areas that can't easily be fixed by heating the area with a hair dryer.
- If one foot is sloppier than the other, see if the store will sell you a half size smaller for that foot. Bonts are sold in different sizes for left and right feet.

Shops that have great reputations for selling ice boots have the years of expertise you want to get the right advice and the proper fit. I've found that most pure in-line stores or general sporting goods stores know very little about boot technology and are so over-whelmed with "moving product" that they aren't much help. I've had good shops really mess up with downright dangerous installa-tions. Remember, this is not a mature technology, so expect to run into some trouble.

Skating puts the most pressure on your feet of any sport. With new or ill-fitting boots you're sure to develop painful blisters. Carry Band-Aids or moleskin and cover up trouble spots early. Be really aggressive about punching out painful areas in boots after heating them with a hair dryer. Alternate new and old boots or cross train while you get used to your new boots.

Think of all those children who appear to skate on the inside of their ankles instead of their blades. There are two big misconceptions about their poor form. First, that they have "weak" ankles. Second, that incredibly stiff boots will fix the problem. In fact, many beginning to intermediate athletes think they need tremendous amounts of ankle support to keep them from caving to the inside or the outside. The real reason the feet cave in or out has little to do with the skater or the amount of ankle support. If your foot can be positioned in an exactly neutral position so that it doesn't cave in or out, little ankle support is required. With the proper alignment, you'll be an ace rather than a clumsy oaf that other kids make fun of. How do you get in a neutral position? Part of it is having a footbed that supports the foot and corrects for a tendency to collapse in or out.

The first step is to try an orthotic. Orthotics should be extremely thin so they don't take up much volume in the boot. You could consider a custom boot, which is guaranteed to fix the problem. A good local shop can get you to either Bont or Paul Marchese, the West Coxsackie, New York, bootmaker who is considered America's best.

Adjustable Frames

The next step to perfect alignment is purchasing highly adjustable frames, or plates, so that you can position your foot in a perfectly neutral position where it rolls to neither the inside nor the outside. I position the front of the frame under my big toe. Some prefer to leave the rear of the frame in the center of the heel for a longer stride. I like to align the rear of the frame with the inside of my boot, making it really easy to get on the outside edge. This amount of adjustment requires having a frame with lots of lateral adjustment or a boot with mounting holes far to the inside of the boot.

Adjustability may seem like a small point, but it is the whole ball game. Getting set up with a neutral foot assures you of a perfect skating stance and much more rapid progression to excellent strokes.

Custom frames are made from high-quality aircraft aluminum, titanium, or a composite of the two, which has little deflection under

> ## Problem Solving
> - Foot collapses to the inside. Move the plate to the inside of your heel and the ball of your foot on the big toe.
> - Foot collapses to the outside. Move the plate to the outside of the ball of the foot on the big toe and the outside of the heel.

pressure. The frames add tremendously to your power and speed, since you have a very firm platform to push off from. The stiffer the frame, the more power you'll get on push-off and the longer your stroke. Shorter plates give you more maneuverability and are about twelve inches long. The longer the frame, the more stable and the faster it will be. Long is fifteen inches for a five-wheeled plate. Watch out for high tech. I once bought a pair of carbon fiber frames. What a mistake! They were as floppy as an old pair of moccasins. Here's my pick of the current frames:

Chargers. These have an amazing amount of side-to-side adjustment with a total span of an inch and a half. This allows you the greatest ability to customize the frame position. I don't like the extremely small wheel-adjustment holes, since they're too easy to strip, as I found when I put the very first screw in. Also, the positioning plates don't work in front, where they are most needed. You can't use the rearmost mounting holes to get the frame as far back as you might like.

I shelled out $240 for this frame and was distressed to find one of my brand-new racing wheels chewed up like someone had taken a lathe to it. One of the mounting screws had no room to clear the wheel. By remounting it one position forward I solved the problem.

Mohema. I bought the standard Mohema frame. It was really stiff and gave a fairly good push-off, but I found two big problems. First, you can't get the plate back as far as you should to get a really good push-off. Second, there's not much side-to-side adjustment. As a consequence my boot would just collapse to the inside, so I looked like a four-year-old. You can mount these frames properly only by redrilling the mounting holes or lucking into a boot that has mounting holes in exactly the right place for you.

Edgemaster. This is a really sweet high-quality frame. But the screw positions on the top prevent it from offering much lateral adjustment. I found I just couldn't get mine far enough to the outside to use. Again, you can redrill holes in your boots for the correct position, but that fixes the frame position, giving you little room for experimentation.

Darkstar. I really love this plate. The four-wheel combination allows you to get close to the ground and still use 80 mm wheels. I discovered, to my dismay, that if you weigh more than 190 pounds, it is just too slow in races. However, I loved its maneuverability and super-comfortable feel. I mounted it with 80 mm Kryptonics wheels.

Faster Wheels

Wheels are the whole game in skating. Slow wheels, you lose; fast wheels, you go like lightning. The technology has a basic trade-off: increase traction and you decrease speed; decrease rolling resistance and your wheels can skitter out from under you. The right mix of traction and rolling resistance is specific to each surface you skate on.

Large. Buy larger wheels for speed. These are best for long strides on a course you can really crank on. A large wheel is considered to be 80 to 82 mm. Because they are bigger, it takes more energy to get them going from a dead stop or after slowing for a corner.

Small. Since the turnover rate is faster for smaller wheels, they get going faster, so you can accelerate faster than with large wheels. They are also more maneuverable around tight corners. If you practice or race on a winding or hilly course and you're good at cornering and accelerating, smaller wheels are better. In the spirit of sports-improvement technology, try the smaller wheels to improve your acceleration and cornering in practice. These measure 76 mm. Even though Americans consider 76 mm small, they are the largest the

Europeans use. If you're on trick skates, you may prefer even smaller wheels to increase maneuverability and deliberately slow yourself down. However, if you are tall like me, an 80 mm wheel is considered small.

Hard. Harder wheels go faster, since they stick less to the pavement, but they can give a very rough ride on less than perfectly smooth surfaces. You want the hardest wheel you can comfortably skate on. Hardness is rated by durometers. The hardest wheels are 82 durometer. If the wheel delivers a ride so rough you can't stride effectively, you need a softer wheel. If you lose too much "bite" into the pavement, so that your wheel skitters, you'll also need to consider a softer wheel. The heavier you are, the harder a wheel you'll want. I weigh 200 pounds and find a 78-durometer wheel soft enough for most surfaces.

Soft. You'll know when you need a softer wheel because your teeth chatter and your eyes dance as you roll over rough pavement. The key is to have a wheel that has a great feel and is still easy to control. You've gone too soft when wheels provide excessive stick. Try several levels of hardness. Clearly, at heavier weights and with fewer wheels on a skate, a harder wheel will feel softer.

Racers are putting harder wheels on the fronts of their skates, where they expect the most wear and where they need the least traction. Since most of your weight is on the back wheels, these can be softer, so you don't slip on corners.

For training, I like a soft, comfortable wheel that has good grip and a nice ride. As you improve your technique, you'll go to harder wheels. As a novice, there's no question but that large, hard wheels will intimidate you, whereas smaller, softer wheels will enhance your learning. Big, hard wheels will shorten your stride and make you feel clumsy.

Shape. The Labeda and Kryptonics wheels have more of a conehead shape, while the Hyper wheel is very round. The conehead shape makes transitions from inside to outside of the wheel very easy to feel. The rounder wheel gives you a more gradual transition.

Core. Manufacturers can put suspension into the wheels so that a very hard, very large wheel can "feel" softer in its ride. I've found that very hard Labeda wheels give a very soft ride because they have a very forgiving hub.

The biggest names in wheels are Labeda, Kryptonics, and Hyper.

Labeda. For my weight, the hardest Labedas ride a great deal softer than the Hypers, so they're a faster, more comfortable wheel.

Kryptonics. The Kryptonics also give a very soft ride for hard wheels. They're excellent wheels for learning. The Kryptonics appear glued to the road and have a very nice feel, but don't seem as fast as Labedas.

Hyper. Hypers have performed extremely well on the race circuit and have the hottest technology behind them. I've found them hard and skittery to race on.

Faster Bearings

Bearings are a critical element for racing. The rotating speed is rated on an international standard called an ABEC scale. The fastest bearings are Swiss. The trade-off is that they must be lubricated more often. For practice I like Bones bearings. Bob Lagunoff of Skatey's Sports in Venice Beach, California, pries off the outer guards of the bearings to cut down on friction and make them even faster. ABEC 1 bearings are the fastest. ABEC 3 is the fastest you'll find in most shops. Bones uses a nylon bearing retainer to make them much less resistant. Most are produced at ABEC 3 and ABEC 5 ratings. These are the easiest to maintain and require just a drop of lubrication. Twincams don't require much maintenance either.

Protective Gear

On speed blades, I always wear protective gear. If you hit a stone, get cut off by a taxi, get run into by a cyclist coming in the other direction, or suffer a wheel blowout, you're going down. With protective gear, you'll go for a controlled slide and then continue skating. Without it, you're laid up for a week or more. I always wear wrist guards. The most common fall is on an outstretched arm, and your wrist or the small bones in your hand are the most likely targets for fracture. Really good knee and elbow pads give you the impetus to go for it. I've found Rector tends to stay on during a long sliding fall, which is what most of them are. You may feel less vulnerable to head injury while blading than cycling, but a helmet does allow you to do a nice roll without fear of cracking your skull. Be careful about the back of your helmet, since in a low aerodynamic position a bike helmet with a swooping tail will prevent you from lifting your head in a low tuck. There are specific helmets for speed skating such as the ones that Flyaway makes.

While you're perfecting your technique the right protective gear can allow you to get much better. The better gear doesn't just work better, it's less obtrusive, looks pretty good, sticks to you when you really need it. Velcro kneepads are a great idea. I can't count the number of times I've put my blades on before I noticed I didn't have my knee pads, then had to take my boots off again! For really un-obtrusive safety gear, look at Trace elbow and knee pads. They're a thin slip-on material. If you don't like clumsy wrist guards, check out Landing Gear. They're lightweight gloves with built-in plastic protectors considered acceptable by the International Skating Association.

GETTING GOOD FAST

Power blading is a wonderful sport in which to think about your technique every time you train. You can change one variable at a time and then watch the effect. For instance, you may lower your body position by getting your thighs into a position more horizontal to the ground. You can practice leg extension simply by straightening your leg. Every time you get on skates, you'll find you're better technically. That's rare in any other sport. This kind of continuous monitoring and improvement makes blading a joy.

Create an Image

Blading instructors are as hard to come by as good racers to model yourself after. Dianne Holum's book, *The Complete Handbook of Speed*

Skating, is a classic sports science text that will paint an exacting picture of perfect form. Special Equipment Company in Acton, Massachusetts, Rollerblade, and New York–based professional in-line skating instructor Joel Rappelfeld (*Get Started in Blading*) all have videotapes. The best technical form is practiced by ice speed skaters, should you have the opportunity to observe them. The basic stroke is slow enough that even an unpracticed eye can pick up a good deal of useful detail.

Get on Your Marks

Blading is the best single sport I've encountered for learning a dynamic athletic stance that can be applied to dozens of other sports. Many men have trouble in sports because they don't have a standard position from which to start learning a sport. In blading, you are motionless long enough at the end of a stride to perfect a balanced stance. You can take this stance into slalom ski racing, Nordic skiing, ice hockey, windsurfing, tennis, you name it. You have excellent markers of your position. Those are very hard to acquire in sports like tennis, figure skating, and diving, where you have to keep track of where you are three-dimensionally in space. With speed skating you're really moving more in two dimensions, so it's easier to keep track of where your limbs are.

Sit on your heels.

Knees no farther forward than your toes.

Relax. Relaxation is such a key part of any sport. Relaxed muscles are more powerful and have greater endurance. In skating they give you added advantage, the ability to react to a fast-changing situation, should you stumble on a stone or have to duck for unexpected traffic. Think of allowing all of your upper-body muscles to lengthen. If you catch yourself "scrunching" up your neck or tightening muscles, think about allowing them to stretch to their longest length.

Lower your center of gravity. By lowering your center of gravity you also create much more stability, plus there's less distance to fall. By getting your knees bent to 90 degrees, you'll gain maximal extension.

If you go lower than 90 degrees, you'll lose power. Speed skaters like to think of this as sitting deeper with the hips. That is, instead of trying to use knee angle as a cue, use your hips as a cue.

Focus your eyes down the track. Look forty to sixty feet in front of you. Looking down will straighten your legs and kill your power.

Align your knees and your toes. The knees should be aligned exactly over your boot during the glide phase.

Learn Cues to Guide You

Glide on a single leg. This is the first goal of beginning skaters to get independent leg action.

Touch your boots. By bringing your boots so close together that they touch, you add length to your stride and facilitate the "fall on your sword" feeling of dropping into your next stride. The biggest give-away that a skater is not that good is when you observe him bringing his feet no closer than eight inches to each other. That vastly shortens the length of the skater's glide.

Stop your arm swing. The arm should really come no farther than across your body and no higher than your nose. Fingertips come to the front of the nose.

Power with your butt. Use the buttocks to press down on the heel of your skate. The buttocks are much more powerful and fatigue resistant than the quads.

Flatten your thighs. There should be a right angle between your thighs and calves. Since the boot tilts you forward several degrees, your thigh won't be exactly perpendicular to the ground, making it difficult to judge when you are in the right position. Trust me that it's unlikely you can hold and maintain this position very long until you've trained sufficiently.

Here's what this extreme degree of knee bend accomplishes. First, you have more leg to extend, so you are increasing power. Second, your balance will improve the lower you go. Third, your air resistance is considerably reduced. Don't expect to go out day one and get your thigh parallel to the ground. Even if you have the strength, you won't have the endurance.

Match your arms to your legs. Dianne Holum coaches skaters to match the legs in force, speed, acceleration, direction, and range of motion with the arms. Both arms are used to accelerate from a standstill. The outside arm is used for cornering and for fast, short courses.

Drive with your hips. Landing on the outside edge of your wheels gives you a longer stride. Don't angulate with your knee. Do bring your hip out to the side past your knee. Your hips should travel in a straight line from one side to the other. Some coaches want you to think of pushing with your hips. Others like the picture of a string pulling your hips from one side to the other. In either case, do learn to push directly to the side with your hips. Many beginners make the mistake of pushing back.

Lower your shoulders to your hips. Your shoulders should be at the same level as your hips. This makes your upper body almost exactly parallel to the ground. This aerodynamic posture will cut the wind as it does for Nordic and Alpine skiers as well as cyclists and ice speed skaters. It provides an enormous decrease in the cost of energy. Try "dropping" your shoulders so you look more like a cat with its back up.

Now here's the tough part. You don't want to bring your head up for two reasons. A raised head increases air resistance and scrunches up the neck muscles to give you a sore neck. That means making an almost straight line along your back, neck, and head. To look forward, you need to lift your eyes as far as possible. Keep your hands in the small of your back and your elbows tucked into the sides of your back for the least wind resistance on long endurance stretches.

Heel down, toe up. During the recovery phase of your stroke, pull your toes up so that your heel is down and you land on your heel. You'll avoid lots of crashes. Try to force the recovering foot at least a half boot length in front of your other foot. That moves your body six or more inches farther forward with each stride.

Land on the back of your skates. Land on mid and rear wheels. The front wheels are like the bow of a ship. The more weight there is up front the more it slows you down. Try putting harder wheels up front as a cue not to get your weight onto your front wheels. By placing the rear wheels down first and bringing the skate down at least a half skate length in front of the other, you'll force the hips down into more of a seated position. That in turn allows for a very long stride, a long glide, and much better power.

Drive your knee into your chest. A great way to get your recovering foot farther forward and keep your back flat to the ground.

Complete the extension. Push to the very end of your stride for maximum power. The extension is to the back at very low speeds, but otherwise should be directly out to the side where you will get maximum bite on the pavement. There should be continuous acceleration throughout your extension. At the end of the extension your knee should be straight and your leg extended as far to the side as possible.

Hold your hips and trunk stable. Your legs need a steady platform to push off from. If you bob up and down, you'll wreck that platform and kill your speed.

Fall on your sword. A fair amount of propulsion comes from just falling onto your new skate. That means moving your hips from one side to the other and not putting your new skate down until you're at the point where you would literally fall and hit the ground if you didn't. If nothing else, be certain that you shift your weight before you put your wheels on the pavement.

Push with your heel. In the basic speed-skating stroke, you push with your heel. Try this and you'll find new power, especially if you're pressing into your heel with your buttocks.

Feel with your feet. The feet are the final common pathway in skating. They give you wonderful feedback on your exact position over your wheel. Pay attention to where the pressure is on your foot. You can experiment with the position of your hips to see where the pressure will end up in your boot. Rather than just thinking, "I've got to be on my outside edge," you can actually pressure the outside rim of your foot and feel the outside of your ankle go into the pocket of the boot. This "foot feel" is magnificent training for Alpine or cross-country skiing, where you get a feel for how you can leverage your skis by changing the pressure on your foot. For instance, you should begin by pressing forward on the front of your boots. You should feel pressure on the balls of your feet. As you go from the outside of your wheels at the beginning of a stroke to the inside at the end, you can feel the pressure shift from the outer edge of your foot into the arch. As you set your skate down on its heel, you can then feel the forward transfer of weight. That sense of foot and leg position is all given to you by just feeling the boot. As cues you have the pressure on the inside and outside of your ankles, the balls or heels of your feet, and your shins on the front of your boots.

Take a straight line on the pavement and try to stay on it. The more your blade angles to the side, the more you'll come off a painted white or yellow line and the more you'll see it weave back and forth under you. Bring your blade so that it is exactly parallel to the line. Use the line as a cue to tell you if you're successful.

Push from the turn. Center your body on the line that describes the turn you are making and then push off perpendicular to that line.

Keep your arms on pins. Dianne Holum coaches her athletes to pretend that their arms are connected by fragile pins to their shoulders. If you do, you'll rotate your upper body much less and won't tighten your neck, shoulder, or back muscles. It's the best arm cue there is.

Widen your stance on fast downhills. By widening your stance on downhills and in corners, you add stability.

Get Good Error Correction

Since good coaches are hard to find, most skaters are self-coached. Since you repeat the same stroke over and over, it's easy to look for errors and correct many on your own. Here are a few to look for:

- Don't drag your front wheels.
- Don't lift your recovery skate too high.
- Don't look down.

- Don't make a circle with your recovery leg.
- Don't dip your shoulders.
- Don't set your blade down in a V. Your wheels should land parallel with your upper body.
- Don't set one skate down next to the other: one should be at least half a boot length ahead of the other.
- Don't tense the upper body.

Play It Back

Skating is a sport that's easily amenable to visual imagery. You can create images that you can play over and over as you fall asleep.

Develop a Checklist

Checklists really work well in skating. Here's a sample list of items to work on while you skate that will really help improve your performance:

- Set your rear wheels down first.
- Push off the middle or heel of the skate.
- Bend your knees to 90 degrees.
- Concentrate your weight on the back half of the skates.
- Keep your arm swing close to your body.
- Stop your hand before it crosses the middle of your body.
- Relax the upper body.
- Drop your shoulders into a cat's back position.
- Tuck in your elbows.
- Look down the track.
- Keep your head level and steady.
- Keep the shoulders parallel to the ground.
- Point your upper body in the direction of travel.
- Keep your hips at the same level throughout the stroke: don't bob!
- Keep your skates close to the ground during recovery.

Remove Physical Impediments

The lower-back muscles and stomach are the real breakthrough muscles to skating fast. In races, sprints, and long-distance workouts in an aerodynamic position, your lower back can tighten like a vise. Only through a combination of training, stretching, and strengthening does your lower back ever get tough enough to handle skating. As recovery declines in your thirties and beyond, the back becomes the Achilles' heel of the sport. The small muscles of the lower back are the weakest link in a skater's entire body. Skaters hang their frames on the small muscles of the lower back. They stabilize their torsos with them while pushing against them with the strongest, most powerful muscles of the body.

What's Dan Jansen's advice about sore backs? "Live with it." While that may be true of Olympic skaters, you don't have to live in pain if you blade for fun and fitness, because you don't have to stay in a deep aerodynamic position to get a workout. I look at blading as an opportunity to develop a terrifically strong back. In fact my back is better now than ever due to the impetus that blading has given me to develop a strong flexible back. As you improve, your back will strengthen. But as it does, lengthening the back muscles, as described in Chapter 26, "Building Elastic Muscle," is the best prevention for lower-back pain.

After a three-mile warm-up, sit down on the ground and grab your frames with your legs fully extended. The warm-up will have made your back much easier to stretch than if you try this before skating, when stretching is more likely to injure it. The incline rowing machine is the best I've found for strengthening the lower back muscles without pouring gasoline on the fire. Roman chair exercising and other trunk-bending exercises can make the back even sorer, since they can irritate the muscle and increase recovery time, which is already the longest for any muscles in the body. The only time your back will really tighten up unavoidably is during a race. If you practice skating with your shoulders and hips at the same level and your trunk parallel to the ground, concentrate on lengthening your neck and back muscles to prevent the natural tendency for them to contract. The more you can extend your neck the better.

Try tightening the abdominal muscles so they are supporting some of the weight of your upper body and actively "pushing" or stretch-

ing out your back as you skate. When you're just starting, cross training is key so that you don't skate every day and over-tighten your
back. Use your hands to knead and massage the lower back in longer
races and workouts.

The performance part of skating is all in the thighs. You have to
hang your entire body weight on one thigh at a time and then push
off with a force far greater than your body weight, like a slalom racer
compressing out of a turn. The extreme angle, with the thigh actually
parallel to the ground, requires tremendous strength on hills. You
will gradually develop that while you skate by lowering yourself several degrees each week. Once you can skate with your thigh nearly
parallel to the ground, you'll develop tremendous power because of
the more extended range of motion you'll have compared to the
average skater, who bends no more than 30 degrees. Stairmasters and
squats are two of the best exercises to get you there. The squats will
build the brute strength to get yourself into a hip-deep position and
keep you there. While the quads are the key power muscles, you're
actually hanging a lot of your weight on your hamstrings during the
glide phase of each stride, which squats will strengthen as well. I like
the leg press machines to build up strength at the extreme end of the
range of motion, because you can lift a high load with a low risk of
injury. With each week you practice, you lower your thighs until
they are parallel to the ground. Building power and endurance in
this position will carry over into a variety of sports from volleyball
and tennis to downhill and Nordic skiing.

Chapter 20

Mountain Biking

AT FIVE O'CLOCK ON A FALL AFTERNOON SEVERAL YEARS AGO, I CHARGED up a long, steep hill in Dover, Massachusetts, on my Charlie Cunningham mountain bike with a twenty-pound knapsack over my shoulders. The handlebar speedometer read 18 mph. Midway up the left-sweeping turn, I saw my prey: a roadie on a $4,500 De Rosa custom bike. There's nothing a mountain biker loves to do more than blow away a roadie (aka road biker). I crept up behind him, then accelerated without giving him a glance. Seconds later, the man on the De Rosa huffed and puffed and slowly tried to blow me away. Determined to sink this Tour de France, Lycra-suited wannabe, I jammed into high gear and blasted past him. Back came the roadie until he was just even with me. As I huffed and puffed and finally blew the man away, I heard him say, "I hope you can do this when you're sixty-nine years old."

Too sheepish to turn around and discover the name of my riding companion, I rode away with a Pyrrhic victory. This guy was tougher than most thirty-year-olds I know. But this same man in a pair of sneakers running up that same hill would have been no contest. Why? The loss of elasticity at age sixty-nine just wouldn't allow him to keep up any kind of competitive speed. But having a great bike is like having a twenty-year-old frame.

A great bike is like an extension of your body. It replaces tired, worn joints and inelastic ligaments. Since you can maintain heart and lung power well into your sixties, the bike becomes a fresh, elastic young new set of ligaments, muscles, and joints. Knowledgeable exercise physiologists call the bicycle the ultimate time machine. Training on a great bike rewards you with a dynamic cardiovascular system, springy, powerful muscles, and the body of a much younger man. Exercise physiologists asked to pick just one piece of exercise equipment for a desert island most frequently select a bicycle. They know they can get strength, speed, endurance, agility, balance, and coordination training all on a single piece of equipment that is also a lot of fun.

> Conventional Wisdom:
> *Bikes are for kids.*
> New Paradigm:
> *Bikes are the ultimate time machine.*

Five years ago only about 20 percent of the members of the U.S. Cycling Federation were forty and older. Now about a third of the membership is over forty.

Mountain Biking Conversion

Manhattan cyclists call it the death ride. Each evening at 7:00 P.M. New York's finest riders meet across from the Tavern on the Green restaurant in Central Park. The best equipment, best bodies, and best outfits on the East Coast mill around at naught point one miles an hour until the last of the traffic clears. The pace is deceptively slow for the first three miles. Then boom, like a man shot out of a cannon, the group sprints the 110th Street hill. Keeping up with the pack, and not behind it, was part of my life in New York for nearly ten years. But one day a new rider blew me away. Instead of a skin-tight Lycra suit, he had on sneakers and cut-offs! Worse, he was passing the pack. But the final humiliation was dumped on the pack by the sizz sizzz sizz side-to-side sound of the knobby protuberances on his tires, which gave away the fact he was riding a mountain bike. I'd give chase and pass him, then he'd pass me, then I'd pass him. Finally, at the end of the evening's ride I introduced myself. The young man, with a modest and pleasant smile, said, "Want to give it a try?"

I had been determined never to ride a mountain bike. I thought they were heavy and slow. To my surprise, his bike was light and fast, yet it could glide over rock, grass, dirt, and sand. After years of seeing life only from the road, my imagination ran wild. Mountains, parks, forests, beaches . . . all could be ridden on a mountain bike. I called up the boys at Sunshine Bikes in Fairfax, California. Could I order an Otis Guy custom bike just like my friend's?

Within a week, the bike arrived. The upright riding position was really comfortable and felt so natural compared with the hobbled-over scrunch of the roadie. The gearing was spectacular. There was no running out of gears to spin on the steepest hills. The bike just sang on uphill sprints. By the next week I'd traded in my Lycra for surfing shorts and a "My other bike is a Cunningham" T-shirt, the Cunningham then being the two-wheel equivalent of a Ferrari. After years of road racing injuries, I'd found my salvation.

Mountain bikes have been called the most fun you can have with your clothes on. They're great adventure vehicles. I've ridden mine in East Africa, throughout the National Parks of the American West, the foothills of Tuscany, along the Thames, and through the streets of New York and Nairobi. The sweet smell of an early morning ride through a slowly waking forest is as great a reward as there is. You'll feel terrific in the here and now. Full suspension systems allow you to descend the gnarliest, bumpiest trails in comfort.

WHY MOUNTAIN BIKE?

Bikes Accommodate the Body Better Than Any Other Piece of Exercise Equipment

Bicycles can be customized to a degree just not possible with any other sports equipment, accommodating any leg, arm, or upper-body length. You can sit upright on a mountain bike or sit back on a recumbent bike rather than scrunch over on a road machine. Crank lengths and multiple gears can accommodate a large variety of different muscle-fiber types from those in the fastest sprinter to those in the slowest endurance rider. There are bikes built to go on snow, ice, dirt, mud, even water. But the biggest advantage is that you can throw yourself on a properly set up bike for any distance, any intensity, and yet run only the tiniest chance of an overuse injury.

Cycling Is the Perfect Sport for Nearly Everyone

Adjustments in frame size and materials mean that anyone can effect a perfect interface between the technology and the body. Strong sprinters can use stiff carbon fiber frames to get maximum zip out of their bikes. Endurance types can take advantage of a titanium frame to dampen vibration for a longer, more comfortable ride. If you don't like scrunching up into a little ball but still want to ride on the road, consider a lightweight mountain bike with road tires so you'll be as fast as the roadies.

You'll Get Great Cross Training

Skiing, Nordic skiing, tennis, and speed skating all benefit from the physical training and bike handling aspects of mountain biking.

SPORTS-IMPROVEMENT TECHNOLOGY

Wheels

In the old days tires and rims were wide in order to be durable and offer some suspension. Because they were wide they were also very heavy; this technology was carried over from the 1950s. With the advent of new materials (e.g., aluminum alloys and Kevlar) and technologies such as finite element analysis (FEA), designers could offer much lighter tires and rims that are more durable. Lighter rims and tires lower rotating weight considerably so you can accelerate more quickly and conserve more energy. Low rotating weight and strength and resistance to sideways deflection are the key ingredients to great wheels. I've made my own and bought mail-order from second-rate mechanics. They were all a source of danger and never-ending frustration. Wheels built by the pros can last for years without maintenance.

Tires

Mountain bike tires have improved dramatically over the last several years. They now offer improved puncture resistance, much lower weight, and increased suppleness. This suppleness along with advanced tread designs makes for better traction (in cornering and climbing) and better compliance (for improved road holding). One of the reasons there are so many choices in tires is that there are so many types of terrain and riding styles. There is no one tire that is best in all situations. However, there are designs that enhance performance on specific terrain. If you're on sandy terrain, you want a tread that is high and spaced fairly close together. On muddy terrain, you want a high tread but much more spacing between each tread so the mud can clean itself out of the tread as you ride. On rocky terrain, you've got more latitude. Here, more than tread design, the important aspect is how gummy the rubber compound is. A bike dealer can help you here. He should have a good sense of what works best on the local terrain.

Skid resistance. One of my worst racing accidents was during a Winter Park, Colorado, race. I came zooming down a hill at Mach 1.0, ready to catch the lead pack. On the shallowest of corners, the bike just left me. I ripped up my side and all the clothing on it. What I look for now in a tire is the ability to resist sliding and rolling. In sand, nothing's going to work well. But on good-quality fire roads and dirt, a tire should give you lots of warning before it skids out.

Low rolling resistance. Big soft tires create a very comfortable but slow ride. Most serious riders pump their tire pressure up to at least 45 pounds. On extremely tortured terrain, they may dump the pressure to 40. By using a low-volume, high-pressure tire without too many knobby protuberances, I get a ride nearly as fast as a road bike on tough off-road terrain.

Rotating Weight

The weight that really counts the most on a bike is weight that rotates, such as pedals, crank arms, tires, wheels, chain rings, and the rear-gear cassette. The lower the rotating weight, the easier it is to accelerate. The most critical rotating weight is in the wheels. I've shaved several pounds off my wheels by going from a 2.6-inch tire and oversize rim to a 1.9-inch tire with a rim almost as small as that of a road bike. A light titanium rear cluster and lightweight pedals and cranks subtract further from the weight that rotates. Here's where light rims and wheels really make a talent enhancement difference. Since light wheels accelerate vastly more quickly than heavy wheels, you will "bump and bust" through uphill sections you'd never otherwise consider. Since smaller tires have much less shock-absorbing capability, the frame needs to absorb more of the shock. A titanium frame's natural compliance allows for a much lighter wheel than a nonsuspended aluminum frame.

Shock Absorption

Frame materials still play a big part in absorbing shock. Aluminum gives a terribly rough ride if you're a heavy rider. Even with front suspension, my aluminum bike felt like a medical device designed to break kidney stones. Steel is heavier but is more subtle on rough terrain. I elected to buy titanium because it offers so much inherent shock absorption. However, a titanium frame can be designed to be either stiff or compliant, depending on the manufacturer.

Most experts consider the technological advances in suspension a huge leap for the sport. If you looked at a mountain bike from six years ago, you'd see that it had no active suspension system. There was a passive system, which consisted of the tires and the human body absorbing shock. Today, many mountain bikes offer you an active suspension system. Now, the tire doesn't need to work as suspension, which allows it to do its job better. Active suspension gives the rider a lot more compliance and usually a huge advantage for handling. According to Rob Vandermark, head of research and development at Merlin Metal Works, a manufacturer of titanium bicycle frames in Cambridge, Massachusetts, "When descending you'll be able to go a lot faster for two reasons. First, suspensions are smoother, so you don't get fatigued as quickly. Second, it keeps the wheels in contact with the ground. That gives you more horsepower and handling advantages. Every time your wheels leave the ground, you're handling decays quickly." Adding rear suspension increases these benefits. The downside to rear suspension is added weight, cost, and increased maintenance. Also, climbing is generally more difficult because suspension systems absorb some of the energy that would normally go toward forward propulsion, unless you have a lock-out feature. Front suspension adds weight, cost, and maintenance, but most people find the ride improvement to be worthwhile.

Frame Technology

Exotic new materials transform the bicycle frame into an extension of your body. A carbon fiber frame will give you new pep and pop on ascents. A titanium frame will dampen out the worst washboard. Lightweight steel frames can sprint you ahead of the pack. But watch out for superstiff frames that can rip you up. They're very hard in corners, through bumps, and over washboardlike fire trails. Very flexible frames will suck energy out of you. You'll have a hard time getting much of a workout, but you will tire. Too much mush doesn't come just from a frame. It can also come from too much "give" in the suspension system, soft tires, and poorly built wheels. Figure out the kind of terrain you'll ride on, then determine where to get your best shock absorption. I found it best to have stiff shocks and a titanium frame that accommodated stiff, light wheels.

Handlebars

Most mountain bikes have straight motorcyclelike handlebars. According to Rob Vandermark, straight handlebars aid in control. "The grip on the straight handlebar is wider apart [than road-type handlebars] and because of this you have better leverage over the front wheel, which makes it easier to steer through rocks and mud and generally increases your handling."

Gears

Whereas four years ago mountain bikes had fifteen or eighteen speeds, today they have twenty-four speeds. Rob Vandermark of Merlin adds, "More gears allow you to have a closer ratio from one gear to the next. This way you can find a really precise and efficient gear for a specific terrain. Your cadence, or your pedaling revolutions per minute, is important to your efficiency, so the closer you can get that to ideal, the better off you are. Extremely low gears give you better leverage to climb short, steep hills."

Brakes

Brakes have a big effect on how fast you go. Vandermark says, "The better your brakes work, the faster you can go — down a hill or into a turn — because you know you can stop quicker." Because you know your brakes are good and you have control, you feel more freedom to take risks. It makes you a more aggressive mountain biker. Brakes have improved drastically. They are better designed and much more sophisticated. On dual-suspension bikes, such as Litespeed's, the frame twists and torques around the suspension points, so the wheels will rub against the brakes unless you set the brakes farther from the rim. If you do, you'll notice that your braking power has effectively been reduced to that of a car on an ice skating rink. Lighter, better disc brakes may be the best solution for fully suspended bikes.

Total Weight

Lots of mass-marketed fitness bikes weigh in at thirty pounds or more. That's a hell of a load to truck up a hill. These supercheap bikes often won't last you through the first week. Below a certain price, you'll spend 50 percent of the bike's cost on repairs in the first year if you ride hard at all. But chances are you won't, because the bike is dull, heavy, and lifeless.

How light is too light? The ad read: twenty-pound dual-suspended titanium mountain bike. Could it be too good to be true? You bet! The titanium bolts that hold the seat to the seat post sheered clean off, leaving my seat on the trail. Several months later, the seat post itself began to break in two. The titanium cogs were too light for steep ascents. The extra pressure on the rear cogs deformed them and pulled the chain clear off the gear. The cranks also were too light, bending and creaking with each pedal stroke. The wheels as well were too light, unable to withstand the side-to-side deflection of tough ascents or the pounding of hair-raising descents. In fact the wheel has a nice crumpled S pattern now. I paid $5,000 for the titanium bike and then another $1,800 to make it rideable.

Be really careful with aftermarket components. Some of the stuff is true space age technology — complete with NASA's track record for equipment failures. Make sure the aftermarket stuff is durable, even if it weighs a few extra ounces.

Stem Length

"If you want to create a further distance between your seat and the handlebars to get you more stretched out, don't move your seat back. Get a longer stem. If you move your seat back, you're affecting your whole biomechanical position over the pedal," advises Ned Overend, a three-time world mountain biking champion.

Pedals

Clipless pedal technology may lend the biggest single advantage to the average rider's power and style. It allows you to get a much better connection to the pedal and to pull up much more forcefully with your foot for added propulsion. Because you are locked in place, power transfers smoothly and you ride more efficiently, with better control. There's also a terrific safety factor. On tough uphills, it's great to know you can always bail out safely should you fail to make it. The best pedal for someone new to the sport is a double-sided pedal. Many beginners get very frustrated with single-sided clipless pedals.

Training Equipment

Bicycle computers coupled with heart-rate monitors allow you to regulate your performance as precisely as a racing car. You can watch instantaneous readouts of speed, cadence, heart rate, altitude, you name it. This means that you can know more exactly what you're doing on a bicycle than any other piece of exercise equipment.

Helmets

A lovely evening ride under a full moon with the smell of salt water in the air . . . jump cut . . . bright overhead lights in an emergency room. Nurses and doctors poke you and ask you questions you can't understand. Accidents happen that quickly. Last year, during the July Fourth weekend, I elected to ride my bike after a long and calorically excessive meal. I didn't have a helmet. I decided to cruise down the bike path the twenty miles to home. I never made it. I woke up in the hospital emergency room. I had been unconscious for a good ten minutes at the scene of a collision between my bike and that of a cyclist who was coming in the opposite direction in the wrong lane. The brakes on my Litespeed Titanium had frozen. It was three hours before I could remember anyone's name or pass a neurologic exam. I had nearly fifty stitches in my head, a major concussion, and retinal damage to my left eye. A policeman at the scene had said, "Nice five-thousand-dollar bike . . . too bad he didn't have a fifty-dollar helmet." The 911 tape said, "This guy looks pretty bad." I wear a helmet now because I know that accidents truly are unpredictable.

How to choose a helmet. Go to a store that has a large selection. Look for the coolest, latest-trick-looking helmets and try them on. They should fit naturally to your head. Some are very awkward and will always feel uncomfortable. Others feel terrific from first hit. Make sure to try the chin strap at the tightness you'll ride with. That brings the front of the helmet securely down onto your forehead. Most helmets are superlight. Make certain there's great ventilation. You're most likely not to use a helmet when it's hottest. There are two separate standards for helmets. ANSI is one, Snell is the other. Snell is a more rigid standard and charges more for its certification. It's worth the extra money. When helmets work, they work wonders.

GETTING GOOD FAST

Create an Image

Ed Pavelka, executive editor at *Bicycling* magazine, says the best way to create an image is to look at photographs. "Sure, we're limited to stationary pictures in the magazine, but readers can study a picture and really break down each body position to learn. The look of the rider sticks in your mind and gives you something that is concrete. We feel it works so well that we've got a section called Riding Technique. We'll have pictures of cyclists descending, climbing, or cornering where they're doing it just right. We'll put a description with it, but I think the words are much less important than the image." Video, says Pavelka, is good if it has slow motion and is instructional. There's not enough time, for example, in a race video to capture, memorize, and reflect back on what to do.

Tim Blumenthal is the executive director of the International Mountain Bicycling Association (IMBA), a group that promotes mountain bike education, specifically how enthusiasts can ride to preserve the land and preserve the experience of other trail users. He believes that going to see and follow a race, on foot, is the best way to get a blueprint for your image.

"There are two racing situations that are particularly instructive. One is steep climbs. If you're standing on the side of the trail watching mountain bikers go up a steep climb, they're moving real slow — 4 or 5 mph — we're talking about climbs that defy the limits of traction and lung capacity. It's really great to see the position on the bike and where the riders' eyes are focused. You get a really sustained look at top racers by standing on climbs at big races. The other thing at races is technical situations like when there are rocks or exposed roots or downed trees across a trail. These are situations that most mountain bikers would say, 'No, way. I'm going to have to walk through this.' You can see the expert racers come through absolutely smooth, relaxed, totally in control. You just watch how they do it. You learn so much technically — how they lift the front wheel up and over objects, how they're really soft on the brakes and

278

just really fluid. There are big races in every part of the country and there's a lot to learn. The secret to watching a mountain bike race is to get out of the start/finish area — where there's not a difference between a road race and a mountain bike race — and go up onto the course, into the woods. You get a real appreciation of their level of skill and daring."

Ned Overend, coach of the Specialized Team and a three-time world champion, says he pictures the act of climbing in mountain biking as a rhythm. "You have so many muscles that work in rhythm together. Your arms are pulling back and your legs are going down and your chest is coming down somewhat. It's a forward, short, rocking motion. The chest and neck are relaxed but the other muscles are contracting." For descending, he says, "The image is your body as a shock absorber. Not fighting bumps, but absorbing them."

Get on Your Marks

Your starting position is largely defined by the way your bike is set up. The seat-to-pedal and seat-to-handlebar distances set you up perfectly or not on your bike. This in large part determines your success at the sport. Poor positioning means discomfort, fatigue, and poor performance.

The standard mountain biking position according to Ed Pavelka would be a lower position with a good amount of bend in the elbows. He adds, "The upper body is further angled forward more toward the handlebar, but balanced; you're not overloading the bar or overloading the saddle. It's a position from which you can do anything. A good rider will almost look as if they're ready to pounce. They're balanced, they're low, they're flexible, nothing is rigid. Their weight is distributed in such a way that if you hit a bump it's not going to make the bike veer or buck."

Ned Overend says there are three biomechanical aspects to the on-your-marks position:

Seat height. "There's no exact seat height for everybody. For example, if you have a long foot, you'll need a higher seat. Also, some people will naturally pedal at the bottom of the pedal stroke, with their heel low, which means your leg will be further extended. You can't require people to pedal in a certain position. There's a range." However, the formula that's most widely accepted is .883 times your inseam — the distance between the bottom bracket spindle and the top of your seat.

Seat position. "You need to adjust the seat forward and back. If you're dropping a pendulum through the bottom of your kneecap, with the pedals parallel to the ground, you want the pendulum to drop through or behind the pedal spindle. What this is doing is setting up this on-your-marks position." For severe climbs and descents, I like to get my weight back to put more weight on the rear wheel.

Position of the ball of your foot. "The ball of your foot should be over the pedal spindle or slightly in front of it. If it's behind, it will create problems with straining the tendons under your toes and in the front of your feet. You also won't have as good a platform for absorbing shock."

Find the Right Stance

Each phase of mountain biking has different stances for uphill, down-hill, standing, or cornering. Here's Ned Overend's best advice.

Uphill. "You should be bent at the waist. Slide forward and back on your saddle to increase weight on your front or back wheel. When your body comes back, it puts your weight on the rear wheel, which helps you get traction. When your body goes forward, the weight goes with it, taking away some of the traction on the rear wheel, but keeping the front wheel on the ground. Often it's a balancing act, moving your body forward and backward with the steepness of the hill. You want to get maximum traction at the rear wheel, but at the same time you don't want your front wheel to start coming out in the air or else you'll lose control for steering. Your arms should be bent, for shock absorption. Pull back with your arms, not up. When you push back, push your torso into the saddle. This will create pressure on your seat and your pedals, which means more traction. Pulling back on the right side of the handlebars as your left leg is going down (and vice versa) creates leverage with your whole body, resulting in increased pedal force. To maintain rear wheel traction, use the bar ends on the handlebars. These were developed to help increase leverage by pulling on them. Think of power flow through your body coming from your hands, through your arms, down through your torso, into the pedal, and then into the ground. It's a line of power."

I've found that bikes set up to spread the rider out lengthwise across the bike are terrific for killer ascents. They allow you to get your butt way back over the rear wheel and still keep your hands way far forward to keep your front wheel on the ground. Long bikes have a long top tube, a long handlebar extension, and a seat that is set as far back as possible. The technique is a very smooth almost relaxed pedal stroke to avoid spinning the rear wheel. Top California rider Austin Hearst pushes his bike forward with each down stroke to avoid spinning the rear wheel. He also pushes the bike over onto firmer, less worn treads for increased bite.

Downhill. Ned says, "Look ahead on the trail to anticipate obstacles. Because you're going faster on the downhill, you should be looking farther ahead than on uphills or flats. You should be standing up with the feet parallel to the ground — the crank arms should be parallel to the ground. The reason for standing is that you want to lower your center of gravity. Standing lowers the center of gravity to your feet and you'll be much more stable. Your arms should be extended but not locked at the elbows. They should be slightly bent to absorb shock. This is because you should be pushing your weight back off of the front wheel. You need your weight back on downhills because if you have your weight on the front wheel and you hit a bump it propels your weight forward and causes you to go over the bars. Your body should be crouched and your butt should be toward the back of the saddle. Your knees should be bent for shock absorption. For the extreme steep on loose, slippery soil, top California riders get their butt in back of the seat and skid the rear wheel while letting the front wheel float."

Standing (pedaling technique on a moderate hill). "You should be standing because you can incorporate more power by using your body weight by pushing down on the pedals and by leveraging your arms against your leg. You leverage your left arm with your right leg and vice versa. You don't want to stand straight up because that will put too much weight forward and take your weight off your rear wheel and you'll lose traction. You will be somewhat bent at the waist. You will be above the saddle, and your butt should be right in front of the saddle, specifically over the bottom bracket. Your arms should be bent. The weight should be over the center of the bike, the bottom bracket. You'll be dropping your weight onto the pedals. Your vision should be straight ahead, but not that far ahead, because you'll be going slower than you will on the downhill," says Ned.

Cornering. The cue here is to lean the bike and not the body. Keep your body straight up to keep your weight on the tires. In a left turn, your right foot is down at the bottom of the pedal stroke. This will stabilize the bike by keeping your center of gravity low. Your arms should be bent. You should be directly over the saddle with your weight equally distributed. You should picture the tire patch. That's the object: to put weight on the tire patch. Think about maximizing the power traction in the turn.

"Search for the right spot to brake by looking for a smooth spot, before the turn, so you can get on that front brake, scrub off some speed, and then get off the brake before you get into the turn," says Ned Overend. "Look where you want to go, not where you're afraid to end up."

Find the Right Cadence

When I was just out of college, I purchased my first really hot racing bike. It was the first time I could really afford a good bike with the right shoes and equipment. One beautiful spring morning, I rode with my friend Rick Grogan. We left Wellesley and began cycling out to Sherborn, Massachusetts. Halfway out, some bike techies blasted past spinning their cranks at 100 rpm. We stood up in our biggest gears to catch up, but at a cadence of only 50 rpm. We found ourselves dusted. That was my first appreciation for the importance of the need to pedal at a high rpm.

The message really hit home several years later when I rode with the great Francesco Moser. At the beginning of a five-hour ride, he had a superfast cadence, about 120 rpm. At the end of a five-hour ride, he still had a superfast cadence. What he taught me was that at any time he could spin up to a sprint, whether it was at the start line or the finish five hours later. A fast cadence gives you the reserve to dig down and "spool up" past other riders. From a physiologist's viewpoint, a low cadence means lots of blood vessels are momentarily shut down during each stroke at high load. This means that legs tire more quickly. You may also be going "anaerobic" before you need to. That depletes your muscles of energy stores very early on. By spreading the load at a higher cadence, you get to actively rest your muscle for when it's really needed.

So what's the ideal cadence? At very low workloads, you can get away with a low cadence, because you're just not doing enough work to wear out your muscles. For the average rider, 70 to 90 rpm is just about perfect. At very high sprinting speeds, you could momentarily go to 120 to 140 rpm. On a mountain bike I'll spin less and "crank" slightly more to get over rubble, loose stones, and sand without spinning. It's the same principle as starting a car on ice in a second gear to get more traction. The ideal way to determine your cadence is with a bicycle computer. Once you've gotten the feel for different speeds, you may look down less, but in different terrains, different distances, states of training, and preparation, you may misjudge your cadence. I usually just count the number of left-hand pedal down strokes in 15 seconds and multiply by four.

Play It Back

Mountain biking has the same rhythm and many of the same muscular movements as downhill skiing. Pick a favorite piece of terrain and ride it over and over until you have it perfect. Then play that back using visualization as you go to sleep.

Learn How You Learn

Better riders really will empower you. "People get into bad habits or get frustrated because they can't do things well, because they're out there alone or they're out there with people of their same ability and there's no model," says Ed Pavelka. "You've got to have a great rider in front of you but also someone that's willing to let you follow them. There's no way they can go at their normal pace — you won't be able to keep up. You will not always make every obstacle. You will fall over or put a foot down. One of the best ways to learn is to go back down the trail and turn back around and try several more times. The next time you come up against something similar, you'll have the confidence."

Remove Physical Impediments

Ed Pavelka says, "At the gym, mountain cyclists will do the typical lower-body exercise — squats, leg presses — to develop more strength. There's a movement in the sport to shy away from leg extensions. If you do a full leg extension, it really puts a load on your knees. That movement is not transferable in cycling. Some doctors are joking that the only time you'll ever use the movement of a leg extension in cycling is when you kick your bike after you've just lost a race. A full leg extension is way past what you need in cycling, and it has been proven to be potentially damaging to the knee. Any time you go out and ride hills, you're giving yourself what's tantamount to lifting weights because it's hard pedaling all the way. Most cyclists feel the best training for cycling is to ride your bike — any bike. Mountain bikers will ride road bikes in their training to gain endurance. You can ride for three or four hours at a time. It gives you the speed and variety. And vice versa — a lot of road riders will ride mountain bikes because it's a good change of pace. A lot of riders will, in effect, do weight workouts on the bicycle by doing big gear intervals, hill climbs, things that put a strain or stress on the muscles as well as the heart and lungs, and this develops the strength for cycling. Weight workouts help to a level, but they're not perfectly related to the pedaling of the bicycle, so people will opt for riding the bike for that kind of strength training and effect.

"Upper-body weight training is done to help counterbalance the development of the lower body. Cycling doesn't do anything for the upper body compared with what it does for the legs. You do pull on the handlebars, maneuver the bike — there are some strains there, and if the upper body has muscle tone, you'll perhaps be a better rider because of it. Most of the weight training is done with lighter weights at higher reps rather than heavier weights because they're not looking for bulk and muscle size as much as they are looking for muscle tone and basic strength."

Tim Blumenthal, who used to be an Alpine ski racer and competitor, believes that cross-country skiing is absolutely ideal for mountain bike training: "The terrain — uphills, downhills, flats — is very similar so the heart-rate pattern is very similar. Some of the technical skills are the same — for example, turning. And as aerobic-capacity sports with anaerobic moments, the two sports are very similar. If you can do it, cross-country skiing is the ideal complement."

Chapter 21

Snow Blading

SWEDISH EXERCISE PHYSIOLOGISTS CALL NORDIC SKIING THE KING OF aerobic sports. Those athletes with the strongest, healthiest hearts are cross-country skiers. Snow blading, or skating on cross-country skis, is the newest form of the thousand-year-old sport, making it really fun and very fast to learn. To many men, snow blading translates into dull plodding. It's gotten that reputation from the original granola set. Dressed in multiple layers of woolen clothing, they carried large backpacks, used thick wooden skis so heavy they couldn't do much more than trudge across the snow, and sported turn-of-the-century Smith brothers' beards.

Today's skaters are a completely different breed. They race in one-piece Lycra suits scorned by the plodders. They have high-topped Alpine boots and extralong carbon fiber poles, and they go like blazes. They can roar downhill at 50+ mph, nip through tight slalom courses, and still zip back uphill. Their sport is like rollerblading on snow, yet with much more elegance and grace. This year, super-high-tech short skis are being introduced that allow anyone to skate beautifully on skis in a matter of hours. By comparison, the classical technique of striding on snow takes many years to perfect.

Conventional Wisdom:

Cross-country skiing is a dull activity practiced by people who live on gorp.

New Paradigm:

Snow blading wraps Alpine skiing and rollerblading into a sport that will inspire you to become a true aerobic animal.

WHY YOU SHOULD SKATE ON SNOW

Quick to Learn

A prototype program at the Royal Gorge Cross Country Ski Resort in Soda Springs, California, has first-time skiers skating up and down hills in an hour using short skis called Revolutions made by Fischer. In a weekend, they are skiing competently on moderate terrain.

Fun

There is more variation to snow blading than Alpine. The Norwegians have twelve different dancelike steps to help navigate every kind of terrain. You can make dynamic turns and even run slalom courses. On a modest descent from the Trapp Family Ski Center summit cabin in Stowe, Vermont, to the base, you can make more turns than in several runs down the Alpine hill.

Fast

Skiers can keep up a 12 to 15 mph pace on the flats and go up to 60 mph on downhills.

Spectacular Scenery

Skis give you access to areas of the country all but closed off to others. Royal Gorge, the largest cross-country area in the world, has magnificent transitions from high wooded forests to open Alpine meadows to jagged mountain summits. On a spring day, you can fly across snow as if it were waxed liquid sand.

Terrific Aerobic Development

Cross-country skiers are so fit that they run the danger of tearing their legs apart if they start jogging at the end of the season. The sport builds an enormous heart-lung engine, far more powerful than is required for running, so skiers may trash unprepared muscles and tendons when they run. Because the workout is spread over so many more muscles than cycling or running, it doesn't feel like half the exertion at the same heart rate.

All-Body Muscular Development

Skating develops the buttocks, thighs, abdominal muscles, triceps, chest, and back.

Develops Great Balance

The dynamic balance in Nordic skating translates to vastly improved balance in speed skating and Alpine skiing.

Makes You a Great Alpine Skier

You get a much better feeling for the proper mechanics of skiing since you have only several pounds of equipment. You'll develop great foot feel, an upright stance, and learn to get your hips forward over your skis.

Looks Cool

Colorful, sleek one-piece suits have the same look as those worn by downhill racers. There is no cooler look in sports.

Burns Calories and Rips Off Fat Faster Than a Surgeon's Knife

A 200-pound man in good condition can burn over 1,600 calories an hour. Rather than burning the 3,500 calories in a pound of fat in a week's worth of running, you burn it off in two hours of high-level skiing.

It's the Fountain of Youth

Maurilio DeZolt led the Italian ski team to an Olympic gold medal in Lillehammer. He was forty-three years old — as old as the fathers of some of his competitors. He beat the best Norwegian team in history. Scandinavian ski racers live five years longer than nonskiers — a stunning difference.

SPORTS-IMPROVEMENT TECHNOLOGY

When skating first began, almost nobody could do it. I remember poling and poling to go nowhere fast when the technique erupted onto the international racing scene in the early 1980s. In fact I raced to the head of the pack of the Blueberry Hill marathon start only to fall off the back as I discovered I really had no idea how to skate uphill. It took skilled racers years to perfect the technique. Now, the talent of these superb national team athletes can be unleashed in mere mortals thanks to high-tech equipment. Jim Fuller of the Vail Ski Center says, "The technology is the technique." Today's novice skiers are better skaters than most of those who raced twelve years ago. Even more than in Alpine skiing, the current technique just was not possible without the technology.

Short Skis

Manufacturers are now perfecting much shorter skis with tremendous ease of use. They scream around corners like the hottest slalom ski and are still stable enough for breathtaking downhills. The secret is making them stiff enough to distribute weight properly without compromising stability or speed. The true short skis are around 147 cm. Some Olympic racers are using an intermediate 188 cm length, far short of the traditional 200 to 205 cm. Fischer has even toyed with a prototype 70 cm ski, just a little over two feet. Instructors like short skis because their students have less ski to deal with on uphills. I find them great on downhills with sharp corners. Rather than having to skid or slow down into the corner so you can step turn through it, a shorter ski makes it certain that you will turn the corner without going into the woods. That lets me come into the corner much faster and with more confidence.

Faster Bases

Speed comes from having a very fast running surface and a perfect distribution of your weight on the snow. Rather than extruding the base, the manufacturer shaves the base off a large block of plastic material like a cheese connoisseur delicately shaving a slice of cheese off a large block. The base is patterned by special bottom-finishing machines in a process called *sintering*.

It pays to find out what part of the block your skis come from. The outer portion of the block, often exposed to ozone and ultra-violet light, is much slower. Some firms use skis made from this material for "seconds" and save bases made from the middle portion for their elite racers. The advantage of this new sintered base is that it is flatter, much more even, and holds wax far better than the extruded base.

Perfect Weight Distribution

Sierra Nordic of Soda Springs, California, has a ski-pressure-testing device that shows how much weight a ski can support. Its rules of thumb are these: For laminate skis, look for a ski that flexes out at 10 percent below your body weight. Say you weigh 200 pounds. It should take only 180 pounds of pressure to flatten a laminate ski completely against the snow. For monocoque skis, look for one that flexes out at 10 percent over body weight. If you don't have the perfect distribution of your weight on the snow, you'll lose speed or stability. Make certain both skis have the same flex. I've seen a difference of more than 80 pounds between two skis in a pair.

Monocoque Skis

Monocoque skis have revolutionized Alpine skiing. They promise to do the same for Nordic skiing. The monocoque design gives tremendous flexibility in the tip and tail but great resistance to twisting. That means that they flow through crud, hold on hard snow, and carve beautifully through corners. These skis truly bring you closer to the biomechanical advantage of the elite skier. Since the tips and tails don't twist, these skis have two big advantages. When skating uphill, the ski doesn't slip downhill or wash out. On downhills, the skis can carve a nice turn instead of continuing in a straight line off the trail and into the woods, an event called railing out. The monocoque design is cheaper than conventional skis to manufacture and allows much more precision in designing a ski with the flex and resistance to twisting that makes it fast and highly maneuverable.

Boots

Nordic boots are a technologic marvel. They are extremely light-weight and comfortable, but still have many of the traits of a great downhill skiing boot. Just five years ago, it was impossible to "V2" an entire race course. V2 is a skating step in which you use both poles to push off one side and then the other, much as downhill racers do at the start gate. With the new boots, an entire moderate 15 km race course can be done V2. These boots have good lateral support for edge-to-edge control, but a soft front-to-back flex. Elite-class racers are now opting for slightly lower cut boots to give them more freedom of motion.

Footbeds

A custom footbed gives a skier stability and power in turns. If your foot collapses too much to the inside, you'll always ski on your edges instead of a flat ski. If your foot rolls to the outside during turns, you'll find your skis constantly washing out. I encourage skiers to buy a custom footbed so their feet are absolutely neutral over their skis. Peterson is a popular model that I've bought for both my down-hill and my cross-country boots. Alpina features a moldable footbed in its new line of boots. Salomon sells a canted binding to get you neutral on your skis.

Poles

These are crisp, lively instruments capable of taking hundreds of pounds of force to propel you down the course with just a tiny amount of bend. High-tech materials like carbon fiber combine stiffness with enough damping to cut vibration. Both Swix and Excel make excellent poles.

A longer pole is best for flat terrain and long downhills. It should be about forehead high. If you do lots of uphills and have many tricky turns like we have in Vermont, a chin-high pole is your best bet, since you can overpower the pole and yet retain the greater maneuverability required of shorter uphill skating strokes. If you never ski classical technique and only skate, you may want to consider special skating poles that have a flat handle across the top for better push-off.

Tracks

Aside from frozen lakes and firm corn snow, skating would be very tough without groomed trails. The snowmobiler, although a natural enemy of the purer-than-thou cross-country skier, lays down some awesome tracks that make lots of the backcountry accessible. Vermont has thousands of miles of trails now thanks to the snowmobile. However, the true joy of the sport rests on highwaylike groomed trails that drive through the heart of America's prettiest country. Great grooming equipment has transformed the sport by allowing skaters to just fly across the landscape. It's worth calling ahead to be certain that the area where you plan to ski has "piston bullies" and other great grooming machinery for skating.

GETTING GOOD FAST

Properly executed Nordic skating on skis is a joy to watch. This is one of the most powerful dynamic sports imaginable. The best way to start building a motor program is to think about how you can best propel yourself.

Create an Image

The ideal image of ski skating is most easily constructed from a good coach. Movements are simple enough to pick up quickly in a detailed demonstration. Videotapes are hard to come by and TV coverage almost nil. I like instructors who race, because they'll have a better understanding of what techniques are the most efficient.

Get on Your Marks

Starting from a basic athletic stance makes everything easy in snow blading. With your knees bent, hips tucked forward, weight centered, eyes looking down the track, head upright, and a relaxed upper body, you'll move easily into each type of step.

The "on your marks" position is in the glide phase of a skating stride. The hips and upper body should be easily balanced directly over the gliding ski. The poles should be parallel to the gliding ski so that all forces are going in the same direction. The hips drive in the direction the ski is traveling. There should be no twisting of the hips, knees, or poles. Everything from your head on down should balance in the direction of the gliding ski. The most common error is to look down at your ski tips. That will make you straighten your legs and stick your butt out. The straight leg makes a ski slide so that you move from a position of weakness. An easy way to align yourself is to think toe, knee, nose. If you glance down, you should see all three in alignment.

Learn Cues to Guide You

The hands lead the hips. Drive through with hands first, get your hips to follow.

Drive forward rather than upward. After you compress your body down over both poles, press your hips forward over your opposite ski without lifting your head up or out of the track. It is the hips that transfer your weight from one ski to the other.

Be light and quick up the hills. When skiing uphill, lift your foot underneath your hip, then place it as far forward as you can, setting your ski down on its outside edge.

Use your feet. Feel your feet to be certain that you are spending as much time as possible on a flat ski.

Be aware of the angle between your skis. This is called the V. Narrow the V when you are going fast. As the terrain gets more difficult, widen the V.

Always keep your hips forward. You can vary pressure on different parts of the ski by applying pressure to the heel, arch, or ball of your foot.

Fight to stay forward. There is a real tendency to get on the back of your foot. As in rollerblading, Nordic skiing is a sport where you can really use your feet to feel where you should be. By staying in the center of your boot or slightly forward on the balls of your feet, you'll stay in command of your skis even in high-speed descents. "F—k it, don't s—t it" is the most popular cue used at Royal Gorge. This pithy slogan is a great way to keep your hips forward rather than allowing them to fall back. The other slogan to remember for driving the hips forward is "Poke holes in doughnuts."

Get Good Error Correction

A good coach should be able to easily spot errors you are making, imitate them, and then show you the correct way. That contrast between right and wrong is much easier for the untrained eye to see than just the correct way.

Tune in to Onboard Feedback

Snow blading is a terrific sport for learning onboard feedback. Terrain changes are usually gradual enough that you can "groove" a skating stride.

Visual. As in downhill skiing, you can plan your line in advance. However, with ski skating you have the widest variety of steps to take of any sport on two feet. By looking up a hill, you can plan transitions from double-poling off both sides to double-poling off one side to staggered pole plants as the hill increases in steepness. For downhills, you can plan a tight line to the inside of the turn like an Alpine downhiller and adjust your body position to stick to it.

In Nordic skiing, you can actually look to see if your skis, poles, arms, legs, and feet are all in the right position and then readjust them if necessary, since you're not usually traveling at a speed where that would be dangerous to do. You can look at your poles to see that they are close to and parallel to your gliding ski. You can look at your foot placement to see that it is close to centerline and as far uphill as possible. You can look at the size of your V or catch yourself from bringing your poles too far up or forward.

I like to look at the beginning and end of a stride to be certain that the pointy part of the hip called the iliac crest is in fact pushing forward down the ski.

Play It Back

Ski skating has a wonderful rhythm that you can play back before you fall asleep, in an airplane, or when stalled in traffic. Use your checklist in each stride to be certain it all fits together.

Make a Checklist

In many sports, it's hard to remember more than a couple of items to work on during practice. With ski skating, try changing your scan every five minutes to a new group of three items.

- Drive hip forward over ski in direction of travel.
- Step up the hill.
- Ride a flat ski.
- Bring feet underneath the hips.
- Feel abdominal muscles compress as if doing crunches.
- Snap triceps at the end of each poling motion.
- Make certain that the poling action is exactly parallel and close to the skis. This is called "framing" the skis.
- Read the terrain ahead of time to offset poling to the left or right.
- Be as relaxed and smooth as possible.
- Don't force yourself.
- Compress legs so that you can spring off leg muscles to be more dynamic.
- Really feel buttocks work on the uphills.
- Try to avoid skidding the skis around corners, so you don't lose control.

Run Through the Gears

Nordic skiing frustrates many beginners because it appears to be so difficult. The arms take an enormous load without any increase in speed. Many men draw the conclusion that any improvement will be impossibly hard. However, just as you wouldn't want to ride up a steep hill in top gear on a bike, that same gearing principle applies to Nordic skiing. There are five gears you use from low to high speed and from steep uphill to flat to steep downhill terrain. They are as follows:

First gear: V skate. This is the easiest stride and can be done up the steepest hills with surprising comfort. Each pole is used independently of the other like duck-footed walking: left pole, right ski; right pole, left ski.

Second gear: V1. Double-pole to one side, recover, and push through with the hips on the other.

Third gear: V2. Double-pole on each side for each skating motion.

Fourth gear: V2 alternate. Double-pole alternating from one side to the other. There should be two skating strides without poles sandwiched between.

Fifth gear: no poles. You're going so fast poling wouldn't do any good. You push off to the side like a speed skater.

As you run through the gears, try bringing a tape along to play at the tempo you would like to develop. It's great motivation and will speed up your strokes.

Learn How You Learn

Most people are doers in skating lessons at the Royal Gorge Cross Country Ski Resort, according to Andrew Hall, the Ski School Director. "But you can always pick engineers in the class who want to analyze everything first," he says. While feeling is the more dominant learning style for beginners, that's not true as they progress. The first time out, most skiers may not know why it works, but can feel that it does. "They'll try what you say but only believe it when they feel it," says Hall. Since the action is not so fast that a student is forced to stick with one style of learning, Nordic skiers rely on the whole range of styles. "Everyone has a little of everything in them," says Hall. "Men who want to learn how to skate are enthusiastic and motivated. Like snowboarding, there's a very fast learning curve. You can get to being really decent within a week."

Remove Physical Impediments

In contrast to Alpine skiing, you really can ski yourself into great shape for Nordic skiing if you just ski. Since many of us are not fortunate enough to live near a ski track all week long, rollerblading, roller skiing, and cycling are reasonable ways to stay in shape for the weekend. In the gym, stair machines can get you in great shape for skating. I like to use them with a duck walk stance, keeping my hips tucked in. This stance will increase your heart rate about ten beats per minute and gives you terrific strength on uphill sections. When you begin, start out on flat or mildly undulating terrain so that you build up aerobic power without killing yourself. Even Olympic teams begin the year on flat courses to get down the technique. Your first days are critical to enjoying the sport, which is why you should concentrate more on learning fun skiing like shooting through a slalom course than just logging miles. The wonderful aspect of snow blading is that it is so varied.

Find a Great Coach

Cross-country skiing is much less of an ego sport than tennis or Alpine skiing. You'll find many instructors pretty willing and able. The best quick test is to have them imitate your errors, show you the correction, and then give you several ready-to-use cues that work. You should make progress through even your first lesson. Try to take your first lessons with short skis like Revolutions or Tempos.

CREATING THE MUSCLES OF YOUTH

Chapter 22

Building Young Muscle

I'M A LIFELONG, SELF-DESCRIBED AEROBIC ANIMAL. I'VE RACED ROWING shells, mountain bikes, road bikes, kayaks, canoes, rollerblades, cross-country skies, and speed skates. I've competed in 500-mile road races, marathons, Iron Man contests, and climbed Himalayan peaks. The people I hang out with have long expressed contempt and disdain for bodybuilders. Regrettably, we made a terrible mistake. If there is a fountain of youth, it is the heavy metal in your local gym. If you undertake only a single new step to regain your youth, build new muscle. This has had the single most profound effect on my physical appearance, performance, and attitude in twenty years. Younger women paid little attention a year ago. I had an unattractive roll of fat around my middle complete with love handles, sloppy posture, and twiglike arms. I was an athlete in attitude, but certainly didn't look like one. Now women who never gave me a look a year ago make offers I haven't heard for years! On the sports front I can do things that I haven't done for decades.

Just a year ago, I couldn't bend my knees to play tennis or ski properly. I felt middle age finally pulling me down and reckoned that the changes were irreversible. I considered surgery on my knees and right shoulder. Now I have explosive leg power and the knees of a twenty-year-old. I've perfected the tennis shots I couldn't do a year ago, because I lacked the power and strength. I can relentlessly attack the steepest, iciest slope run after run. I have a vastly improved metabolism, which keeps my energy high all day long and keeps fat from creeping around my midsection. If I gain fat over a long holiday, it's gone in a week. I feel that I've shed twenty years.

Conventional Wisdom:
Regular aerobic exercise is all you need to remain young.
New Paradigm:
Muscle is youth.

What can you do about muscle loss? In a major policy shift, the American College of Sports Medicine now recommends weight training for every adult. The earlier you start weight training, the more muscle you'll keep into old age. It's a use-it-or-lose-it phenomenon.

Weight training is also a terrific area in which to practice mental imagery. You can imagine your muscles getting firmer, harder, and bigger. Imaging expert Dr. Martin Rossman, the co-director of the Academy for Guided Imagery in Mill Valley, California, recommends imagining proteins, minerals, and vitamins coursing through your arteries into muscles, providing rich nutrients for muscle growth.

WHAT BUILDING YOUNG MUSCLE WILL DO FOR YOU

Speed Up Your Metabolism

Are these complaints familiar?

- "My metabolism is slowing down."
- "I can't eat as much as I used to without getting fat."
- "My muscle turns into fat."
- "I don't have as much energy anymore."
- "It's harder every year to keep going at the same pace."

These complaints all have a simple explanation: muscles shrink as you age. A big muscle is like a big car engine. Even at idle, big active muscles burn calories. Less muscle causes your metabolism to fall. Dr. Bill Evans, director of the Noll Physiological Research Center at Pennsylvania State University and a top expert on exercise and aging, says, "We feel that older people's reduced muscle size is almost wholly responsible for the gradual reduction of their basal metabolic rate." Metabolism drops 2 percent each decade starting at age twenty.

Recapture Lost Youth

Weight training can wind back the years by giving you the same amount of muscle you had as a twenty-year-old. Unless you were a champion bodybuilder, you can build even more muscle now than you had when you were in college. Research shows that big gains in muscle mass can be acquired until age sixty, moderate amounts until age one hundred! You might think that the idea of young muscle is just figurative. In fact, if you look at the turnover rate of proteins and the other structural components of muscle, you'll find that muscle is completely rebuilt at least several times a year. So even at the age of eighty, well-trained muscle is really young.

Increase Potency

Muscle cuts right to the core of being male. As a man, the fatter you are, the less male sex hormone testosterone is available to your body. The leaner you are, the more testosterone there is to go around and the greater your potency. Weight training increases testosterone availability even in middle-aged men. The combination of increased production and decreased fat is the best natural method of increasing potency. While aerobic training can decrease testosterone production, weight training increases it.

Lower Blood Sugar

Muscle loss may accelerate the speed at which we age. As the muscle mass shrinks, blood sugar levels can increase even without diabetes. These high levels of blood sugar actually cause our bodies to age. They do that damage by attacking the connective tissue in our skin, joints, ligaments, and bones. Connective tissue can be thought of as the glue that holds us together. By age seventy, 20 percent of men have an abnormally high level of sugar in the blood after a big sugary meal. Why is the sugar level higher? Muscle is the primary place the body puts the sugar you eat. If you're active, that sugar is burned by muscle immediately or stored as reserve fuel. If you're sedentary, sugar is circulated back to the liver and converted into fat. As a person becomes fatter and less muscular, insulin, the hormone that regulates blood sugar, doesn't work as well. So as you get older, fatter, and less muscular, your blood sugar may rise.

Increase Energy

How does muscle size affect your energy and vitality? Muscles are a key storage area for sugar. Sugar is stored in the muscle as glycogen. Glycogen stores are limited by the size and conditioning of muscles. Middle-aged men with less muscle can store less glycogen, so they have less energy and less endurance.

Strengthen Bones

Weight training increases bone weight and density more than swimming or running. Since it stresses most major bones in the body, it offers tremendous protection against the thinning of bone known as osteoporosis. If osteoporosis is not as well known as a threat to men as to women, it is simply because men get it at a later age.

Improve Sports Performance

I've been terrifically impressed by how much better I perform in all sports with weight training. Certain muscles are critical to sport. For instance, tennis power is improved 35 percent by an increase in shoulder strength. You're lost without dynamic thigh strength in skiing. The small muscles of the lower back are the weak point of any speed skater or rollerblader. And weight training has been proven to increase motor performance.

Harden Joints

Build muscle to protect joints. Good personal trainers first seek to "stabilize the joint" before loading the muscle around it as a way of preventing injury. For instance, squats will "harden" the knee joint by building much stronger, bigger ligaments and muscles. This strengthened joint develops immunity to routine injuries. The attachment of ligament and tendon to bone, where many injuries occur, also becomes hardened. A big part of staying young is being able to withstand the joint strain of aerobic training and the sports in which you wish to excel. The right weight training will help you do that.

Improve Your Appearance

There is no better solution for the slouch-shouldered, potbellied, bent-over look of approaching middle age than an increase in muscle mass. Men who spend even forty minutes a week weight training have a more commanding presence and more imposing bearing than those who don't. Want to look like a leader? Take up weight training. Adding muscle takes away the urgency to be superslim. Too many men think they'll improve their appearance by stripping off every last ounce of fat. That leaves many of them looking tired, haggard, and old. The skin drapes poorly on their face, their posture is slumped, and the startling loss of muscle mass associated with dieting creates an alarming aging effect.

Lose Fat

Most good research papers show that lean body mass increases as body fat decreases. Because these two changes occur simultaneously, the result is little or no change in total body weight. That's important for aerobic athletes who don't want to gain weight.

Control Your Life

I asked the editors of *Men's Health* magazine why they ran so many articles on bodybuilding. Here's what they said: "Men don't control much in their lives any more. There's not much they can change. Even if you're President there's not a lot you can accomplish. Short of radical plastic surgery, weight lifting gives you tremendous control over how you look." Muscles do get bigger, your posture straightens, the bulges go away. It's something you can do for yourself that achieves fast, gratifying results.

WHAT REALLY WORKS

Building and maintaining the biggest active muscle mass you can is your best way to roll back the clock. In six months, you'll have built enough new muscle to achieve that goal.

The big upper-body muscles you clearly want to focus on are the latissimus dorsi and the pectorals. The big lower-body muscles are the quadriceps, the hamstrings, and the gluteus maximus. Dr. Bill Evans says, "If you're going to be doing specific exercises to prevent losses in muscle, you might as well go for the large muscle groups. You'll get a lot more bang for your buck so to speak."

All muscles have an equally high metabolic rate. By preserving the large muscles, you're preserving more of your metabolic rate. The good news is that these muscles are very easy to build up quickly. As opposed to the endless open-ended commitment that bodybuilders make to weight training, you can hone in on exactly what you want and achieve it in a short period of time.

Even a man in his forties will feel an age-related loss of function. It's harder to lift a box up overhead onto a shelf, squat to lift a load with your thighs, or use your back in sports without coming home sore and stiff at day's end. It's this continuing decline in just a very few muscle groups that eventually makes us frail. In the lower body, those muscles are the quadriceps, hip extensors, hamstrings, buttocks, and muscles that support the spine. In the upper body, they are the deltoids, biceps, and triceps. "The deltoids," says Evans, "are important to a whole host of functional capacities of the arm." These muscles are highly important for prevention of injury and improvement of performance in sports. In tennis, for example, there's a lot of evidence that strengthening the arm and shoulder muscles will help men in their forties and fifties maintain their strength and their game. Coaches who train tennis players are having them do much more weight conditioning than ever before of the biceps, triceps, and deltoid muscles.

All of these anti-aging and anti-frailty muscle groups are very easy to work with and strengthen. Contrast them to the calves or forearms, which take tremendous effort over years to really develop. The muscles needed to reverse aging are truly easy to develop.

WHAT TO EXPECT

Even at age one hundred you can expect rapid changes to occur within the first two weeks of resistance weight training. During that time your brain is making new connections to muscle. The wiring of your nervous system is reorganized so that it can direct your muscles to lift more weight much more efficiently. It's also tapping new parts of the muscle that may have fallen idle. Men under sixty will find by the six-week mark that their muscles are harder and better defined. By twelve weeks, you'll start to "pop" with new hard bulges in places you never thought you'd see them. Progress is very rapid during this time as you lift heavier and heavier weights with less and less effort. A day will come, however, when the progress stops. That's when you know you have to change strategies by incorporating different exercises to stimulate the muscle to grow. These are ingenious and have been worked out by trial and error over the last several decades. Then your progress will zoom again. You'll learn to plan in advance so you don't hit plateaus.

The majority of those who begin a weight training program drop out because of discomfort or lack of results. Here's the good news. Every time you train, you are making much higher quality protein in your muscles, stronger bones, thicker, more shock absorbent joints, and tendons capable of handling much greater loads. This break-in period is just that. Don't let anyone push you in over your head! Lots of discomfort and little progress turned me off serious weight training for decades. The gyms I joined had a complimentary trainer who took me through a sample session. I struggled and pushed and pulled to get the weights to move. My joints and tendons hurt more than my muscle. In retrospect I'm sure I was lifting too much weight too early, not getting the protein I needed to make new muscle, and using machines that just weren't built quite right to prevent joint and tendon pain. With my latest and finally successful attempt at building muscle, I found no pain or discomfort. I made nice progress through all the early stages by doing lots of repetitions and hitting my muscles from lots of different directions. It's critical not to get turned off at this stage, to take it easy enough to enjoy the workouts without expecting huge eye-popping muscles the first week. Your patience will be rewarded.

Since I've made every mistake in the book, here's what I would have done differently if I could start again.

• I would have started slower. In my eagerness to make big gains I tried to push the weight up quickly day to day until I was really yanking on tendons and ligaments before they were ready for the load. Smaller increases in weight would have been more sensible.
• I would have learned strict form at the beginning without trying to "cheat." By lifting big weights too quickly, you have to cheat on form. In the long term, this hurts, since you're not directly stimulating the muscle you want to grow but accessory muscles around it that help you cheat. Any good bodybuilder will tell you that it's the volume of training in good form that counts, not the absolute weight.

Chances are pretty good that if you've read this far, you're a "hard gainer." Most of us are. Even those who made easy gains in their twenties will find them more difficult in their thirties and genuinely hard in their forties. But that doesn't mean it's impossible. It requires maximizing the body's drive to build new muscle. There is a formula that I, one of the hardest gainers, have tried, and it really works.

• Maximize your protein intake.
• Use the best-technology weight training equipment.
• Hit your muscle from several different angles.
• "Periodize" for maximum effectiveness by changing the intensity of your workout at regular intervals.

Genetic endowment determines whether you have large, powerful, "fast-twitch" fibers that easily grow in size with weight training or smaller endurance fibers that are hell to push to any increase in size. Genetics also determines the number of fibers you have and the length of your muscles. Longer muscles can usually develop greater volume than shorter muscles.

If you're a super-endurance athlete with long tendons and short muscles, you have the worst natural endowment for building muscle. Your endurance muscle fiber will be hard to increase in size. The short length of your muscle also decreases the potential for ultimate growth. Chances are that you don't want to become big and bulky anyway. However, you can make enough young muscle to increase your youth.

If you have very long muscles and are a natural sprinter, you have the best combination for gaining weight. You can build a substantial amount of new muscle and then decide at what point you no longer want to gain any more. Remember, the key is not to build lots of extra muscle, but to build enough to turn back the clock. If you look at muscle magazines and wonder why you can't look like that, wonder no longer. Many professionals take anabolic steroids that give them gains that natural bodybuilders can never achieve. Since the point of building new muscle is to regain lost youth, anabolic steroids don't make much sense. They increase your risk of heart disease and liver cancer.

Some men have a fear of building too much muscle. If you're over thirty-five, fear not. You'll be hard put to build more than twelve pounds a year. That gives you ample opportunity to stop when you want. Remember that twelve pounds is regaining two decades of lost youth! How much muscle do you want? First, you want to replace any muscle you've lost. That means returning to the muscle mass of a twenty-five-year-old. Second, you want enough muscle to handle your body weight adequately. Squats, pull-ups, and triceps dips are excellent indicators of that ability. Third, you want enough to bring your metabolic engine to full tilt. Fourth, you want enough strength for sports performance. Any more muscle is wasted. You might be confused by recent reports that men who weigh less live longer. Keep in mind that the study by Stanford University's Dr. Ralph

Paffenbarger did not look at the amount of fat or muscle these men had. The risk is for more fat, not muscle. Also keep in mind that most men will be trading muscle for fat and will end up on the lean side of normal weight. You do not need massive bodybuilding bulk to build youth. Even bodybuilders don't weigh as much as you think. They look spectacularly well developed because they have so little fat to hide their muscle.

Since most men aren't going to embark on a midlife bodybuilding career, I favor spending six months of intense muscle building during which, research shows, you'll increase your strength by 50 percent. At that point reassess the amount of time you can put into training. Most men don't have the time, patience, or dedication to continue building after the initial quick gains and don't really have to in order to gain youth. My own belief is that most men will be very pleased with a well-thought-out six-month training program. If weight training has been too time-consuming, you can cut back and simply maintain what you have. One study showed you can maintain weight training as little as once every two weeks. I favor keeping up a core weight training program twice a week once you've got what you want. For the sake of novelty you can rotate through different muscle groups during the year. For instance, you may favor your quads, hamstring, abdominal, and buttocks muscles before ski season and your shoulder, chest, and arm muscles before tennis season.

Once strength and muscle-mass gains slow, you face a decision. You can accept that you're nearing your natural limit for that muscle and move on to develop other muscles. Alternately, you can change exercises so you hit the muscles from different directions and change the kind of sets you're doing to get a new training effect.

It's very difficult to see the results of endurance training unless you're using a stopwatch. Weight training produces results that are easy to see and feel. Those results will become more striking if you keep a simple log of your results. Here are some observations to keep you excited about your progress:

Phase One: First Six Weeks

- Lifting more weight.
- Muscles are harder.
- Weights seem easier.
- Body fat may be dropping.

Phase Two: Six Weeks to Six Months

- Muscles are bigger.
- Muscle definition is improved.
- Waist is trimmer.
- Body fat is decreasing.
- You can handle much bigger loads.
- Your game has improved in sports.

Chapter 23

How to Grow New Muscle Fast

IS THERE A SPARK OF ENVY AT THE GYM OR BEACH WHEN YOU SEE some heavily muscled young man or woman who seems to have gotten that way almost effortlessly. Do you pump at the gym endlessly with little to show but a little extra tone? ("Tone" is defined as failed bodybuilding.) What have they got that you're missing? It's called the anabolic drive and refers to a constellation of forces in the body that builds new muscle. The anabolic drive helps build bigger muscles, improve potency, and increase sex drive.

> Conventional Wisdom:
> *Building muscle is awesomely hard unless you're naturally endowed.*
> New Paradigm:
> *High-tech training can build all the muscle you need to stay young quickly and effectively.*

HOW TO INCREASE ANABOLIC DRIVE

Use High Resistance

I've had my fill of weight training that won't work. Almost every day a new system of on-the-road or home weight training is advertised on TV or in magazines that couldn't possibly produce the results that the carefully selected models display. We're meant to believe that a shoelace or plastic tube or complicated series of elastics will give you great results. No way!

If there's one solid research conclusion you can take to the bank, it is that high intensity really works. The big breakthrough in weight training for older Americans was the discovery that high resistance produced astounding results, even at age 101! Many men who have never undertaken weight training are put off by the idea of high-intensity weights. However, properly performed, there is no great pain or risk of injury.

Learn Perfect Form

There is no harder tendency to overcome in weight training than the urge to pile on more and more weight even though the exercise is poorly performed. Many novice bodybuilders are disappointed that big bulging muscles don't pop out on day one. But if you use those early weeks to just learn the right movements without being concerned about gains, you'll make enormous progress in the long run. To really push your muscle hard you first need to train or strengthen the levers that control those muscles. Those levers are tendons, ligaments, and nerves. Once those connecting structures are strong as steel, you'll accomplish wonders. Every twinge, ache, and pain I incurred weight lifting I got from poor form. The most compelling reason for good form is that only then are you truly isolating the muscles you want to grow rather than working around them with accessory muscles that don't count for much. Build up to high-resistance weights only after you've learned perfect form.

Go for Volume

Power-lifters do a very small volume of training and it shows. They have a small fraction of the muscular development that you see in bodybuilders. You can lift an extremely heavy weight a few times, and little growth will occur. The great secret of many successful bodybuilders is not that they lift incredibly heavy weights a few times, but rather that they lift moderately heavy weights many times. Volume is measured as the total number of repetitions that you perform of a single exercise. For instance, you might do four sets of eight repetitions for a total volume of thirty-two repetitions. Now, if you do four separate exercises for the same body part, you would perform 128 repetitions, a terrific stimulus for growth.

Go to Failure

Every personal trainer worth his salt will push you to failure on every set. What does that do? Curiously, after millennia of bodybuilding and a century of scientific inquiry, no one knows exactly what it is that causes a muscle to grow. There are several different theories. The acid theory says that you build up enough lactic acid inside the muscle cell to stimulate it to grow. The nerve failure theory says that with multiple sets to failure, you are forcing your body to dig deeper and deeper into previously unused muscle that is then forced to grow. The injured muscle theory hypothesizes that heavy weights cause the muscle to split apart into new muscle fibers, which account for the increased size. All these theories have at their core the need to make a muscle fail so that your last repetition in each set is truly the last one you can do.

Go for the Pump

For every muscle group, it's important to do a set that "pumps" the muscle. That set is performed with lower weight so more repetitions can be achieved. The muscle actually feels larger because it is engorged with blood. For example, you might do two sets of eight repetitions followed by one set of sixteen repetitions. Pumping the muscle gets more blood around the muscle fibers by building more capillaries. Those small blood vessels can quickly take away waste products and transport vital nutrients to the muscle.

Hit the Muscle Every Way You Can

This is the best single way to get spectacular early results. Here's what I mean. You may do a bench press to develop your pectorals. No matter how many you do, you're stimulating only the middle and the center of the muscle. But you can also get the outside, top, and bottom of the muscle to grow by hitting the muscle from those different directions. If you've never weight trained before or had little success, this is the best single way to develop quickly and easily.

Take the Easy Way First

It makes little sense to spend hours trying to build up a calf muscle that just won't budge, when you can make enormous and strikingly easy gains building up your chest, arms, or back. Once you've made gains in the "easy" muscles, you can go for the harder ones, since you will have built the levers of power needed to get at them. You will also have created an enormous muscle-building drive to get at those hard-to-develop muscles by the time you're ready for them.

Start with High-Tech Equipment

Free weights are a great stumbling block to progress when men begin weight training or pick it up seriously for the first time. The extra effort spent learning to handle and balance weights discourages many men. Adding and subtracting weights until you've got just the right amount is very time-consuming. With high-tech machines, you just plug and play. I can move through twenty different machines in thirty minutes where it would take nearly two hours with free weights. Changing weights takes seconds. If the weight isn't just right, you don't have to get up, lift off the old weights, and put on the new ones. High-tech machines give you an instant expertise, because they direct you through the proper range of motion for an exercise. The best machines hit each muscle precisely where it extracts the best training effect. They're a great example of talent enhancement technology. Nautilus led the equipment revolution. Cybex is, in my opinion, the current leader. Its machines are designed from a thorough knowledge of muscle structure, function, and biomechanics. Other machines, which use hydraulics instead of weights, have gained great popularity among older men since they pose little risk of injury.

Progress to Free Weights

Free weights are terrific when you're ready for them. Once you've stopped achieving big improvements on machines, it's time to move on. You'll appreciate how the same exercise with free weights "hits" the muscle in a different way so that you get renewed growth and development. At the point you're ready for free weights, you can decrease the number of exercises you're doing while making great new gains.

Periodize from the Start

Muscles are a lot smarter than they look. They can't be tricked into growing in just one way for very long. Do the same exercise with the same number of reps and sets day in day out, and in several months you'll find yourself stale and your muscle in arrested development. By planning from the start to vary your workouts, you'll avoid that staleness factor. The most important variation is from one month to the next. It's also the easiest to plan for. At the beginning of each month, change the number of reps you do in each set.

Start with Simple Exercises

Early in weight training, joints, ligaments, and tendons are all vulnerable. When performing complex exercises that use several joints, it's difficult to adhere to perfect form because the underlying muscles required aren't all developed enough. Here's a good example. An overhead press is a terrific exercise for the muscles of the shoulder if you are injury-free. However, it is awkward and difficult for a beginner to perform properly. Most men want results, not endless corrections on proper form. I feel it's better to use machines to gain strength in individual muscles first. That builds the strength, coordination, and confidence to progress. Simple exercises also prevent cheating on form.

Progress to Compound Exercises

The more experienced and stronger you are, the more compound exercises you can do. A compound exercise is one that involves muscle groups on either side of at least one joint. When you're ready for them, they're the best of all exercises, because they maximally stimulate new growth and they can deliver huge gains to sport-specific activities. Since complex exercises develop many muscle groups at once, they cut down on the number of exercises you need to do. So, as you get better, you can choose much more efficient exercises.

A squat is a perfect example, because it develops the buttocks, hamstrings, quads, calves, and muscles of the lower back all at one time. That stimulates terrific growth and tremendous crossover power for skiing, tennis, cycling, and a range of other sports. Squats replace individual machines that exercise the quads, the hamstrings, the lower back, and the calves. But if you begin with squats, you'll find them cumbersome, uncomfortable, and potentially dangerous.

Do Weight That Allows Complete Range of Motion

In the rush to lift more and more weight, there is a tendency to complete less than the full range of motion. In the long run you will eventually have to back down to lower weights to "push through" with proper form. A complete range of motion allows you to build up the weakest parts of your muscle so that you can progress.

Do a Balanced Workout

Most men self-select the muscles they are going to develop. These are usually the ones most likely to pop out from under a T-shirt, usually the pectorals and the biceps. To build lots more young muscle, develop the opposing muscle group as well. For instance, the triceps actually builds a much bigger muscle than the biceps. The latissimus build much more volume than the pectorals. Balanced workouts give you a huge expanse of fresh young muscle to develop. It's critical to balance the power in opposing groups of muscles, since a very weak opposing muscle group is prone to serious injury. In the NFL years ago, researchers found that players with dramatically weaker hamstrings than quadriceps had more hamstring pulls and tears.

The most likely imbalance in weight training is between the chest and the back. You can't see the back muscles, and so they tend to be ignored. If you find you have lots of backaches and pains that are aggravated by weight training, take the time out to train your back up to the same level as your chest. Training back muscles is a great way of unloading the stresses of everyday life that tense and cramp back muscles. Once they are strong and supple they are far more stress resistant. Some experts recommend training opposing groups at the same time. That is, do a set that pushes followed by a set that pulls. You can mix biceps with triceps, bench presses with lat pull-downs, leg extensions with hamstrings.

Forget Calisthenics

World-famous athlete Herschel Walker has made calisthenics famous again. He gets the same remarkable results with hundreds of repetitions of calisthenics that bodybuilders do with weights. You, too, can have a great body doing calisthenics, but remember several points. First, you must do hundreds of repetitions. Second, that takes enormous self-discipline. Third, until they have done weight training, many men can't do enough calisthenics to make any progress. For instance, they may get stuck at sixteen push-ups. Without doing accessory exercises, they just never do any more. If calisthenics really worked well, you would have seen millions of muscle men emerge from high school gym classes in the 1950s and 1960s.

Allow Maximal Recovery

There is a new push to train each major muscle group just once a week so that you get maximal recovery. For instance, the quads and lower back recover very slowly, so you could get by with one squat day and one lower-back day. Give big muscles such as the pectorals and latissimus 48 to 82 hours to recover. Biceps and triceps can do with less. Abdominal muscles can be trained daily.

Chapter 24

The Muscles of Youth

MEN DEVELOP CERTAIN MUSCLES FOR A HOST OF PECULIAR REASONS. The bench press is a key locker room status symbol. If you bench-press 220 pounds, it's a big deal. The Popeye image of a strong man features bulging forearms. Chest and calf muscles have become so critical to success in bodybuilding that Beverly Hills plastic surgeons now offer implants for men who are genetically underprivileged or who don't want to spend the time developing them. But to turn back the clock, you need to develop those muscles that keep you young. Those are the muscles of the shoulder, back, chest, upper arms, abdomen, and thighs.

SHOULDERS

Many men stick with biceps, pectorals, abdominals, and thighs for weight training. By adding shoulders, you'll add young muscle that's critical to preventing injury and performing well at dozens of sports, including tennis, baseball, golf, and cross-country skiing. Under-developed shoulders are very vulnerable to injury, since so much power and velocity must be generated by these muscles. Here are the anti-aging individual muscles of the shoulders and the exercises that best build them.

Deltoids

While many men have strong biceps and triceps, the weak link is the deltoids, which can prohibit men from using their strength whenever they lift their arms up toward shoulder level or above. With these exercises, you can develop a moderate amount of bulk in a four-month training program. Serious bodybuilders can build considerable bulk in the deltoids, rivaling the biceps.

Lateral raise. This can be performed with dumbbells or a machine. I prefer the Cybex deltoid machine. It sets you up at just the right angles and is very easy on the shoulders. You needn't come any higher than the shoulder for a good workout. Past the shoulders and you'll begin working the neck. Even if you have a sore or injured shoulder, these deltoid raises can be soothing and a quick muscle builder.

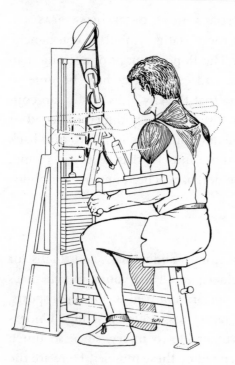

24–1. Lateral Raise

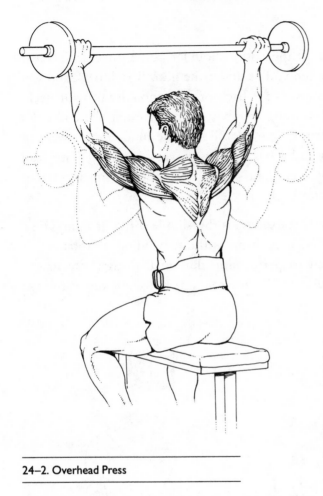

24–2. Overhead Press

Overhead press. I don't like overhead press machines for this exercise because it's too easy to pinch your shoulder and stress it the wrong way. I got so sore and developed so much crunching in my shoulders on an overhead press machine that I could barely play tennis. A simple overhead press with a barbell is extremely gratifying and much easier on the shoulders. The weights need not be very heavy. You can start in the range of twelve to fifteen reps. If you do these presses behind your neck, you'll develop the front and side deltoids. However, the behind-the-head press should be avoided, especially with heavy weights, if you have a torn rotator cuff.

Trapezius

Since these muscles lift the entire shoulder girdle, they are primed for stress. Try this when you're under the gun. Reach back and feel the muscle that runs across the back of your shoulder to your neck. Is it tight and hard? Nothing feels better than working these muscles to purge the stress from them. You'll become much more aware of them and they'll hurt a lot less after just a week's training. They can thicken and develop some anti-aging bulk but are small potatoes compared to the major back muscles, the lats.

Dumbbell shrug. The best exercise is this simple shrug. It should be a straight up and then down shrug without bending or rotation. If you're unaccustomed to performing dumbbell shrugs, stay in the range of ten to twelve reps since too much weight too early can injure the muscle.

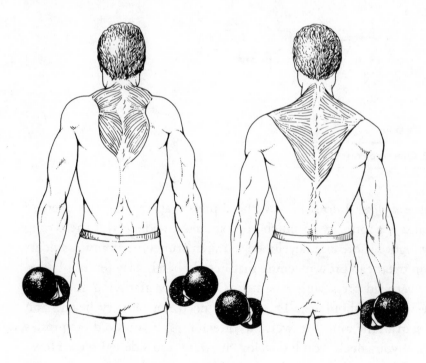

24–3. Dumbbell Shrug

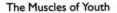

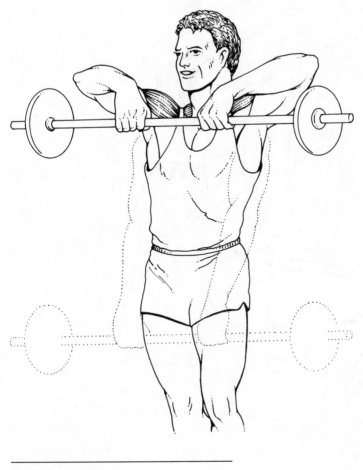

24–4. Upright Row

Upright row. This is an easy at home or gym exercise with a barbell. Avoid upright rows if you already have a bad shoulder, especially a torn rotator cuff. Upright rows can cause or worsen a rotator cuff or impingement problem.

CHEST

The pure bulk of the chest or pectoralis muscles make them key muscles of youth. The pectorals are unique in that they can be hit so effectively from so many different directions for terrific development.

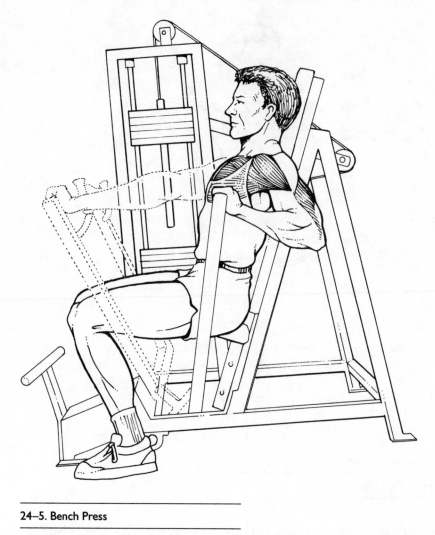

24–5. Bench Press

Bench press. Since the bench press also develops the triceps and front deltoids, it is a super-efficiency exercise for men short on time. If you can do just one chest exercise, do the bench press until development slows. Once you have stopped making big gains with a bench press, you can still make huge gains by developing the upper, inner, and lower pecs.

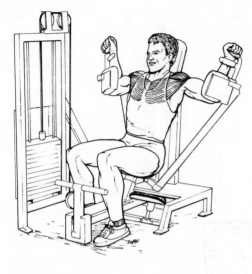

24–6. Fly

Fly. In combination with the bench press, this is a terrific mass builder.

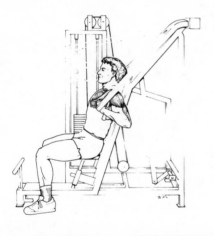

24–7. Incline Press

Incline press. Develops the upper pectorals, which are a great new area to increase in size if you've always stuck with bench presses. Stay away if you have a rotator cuff problem.

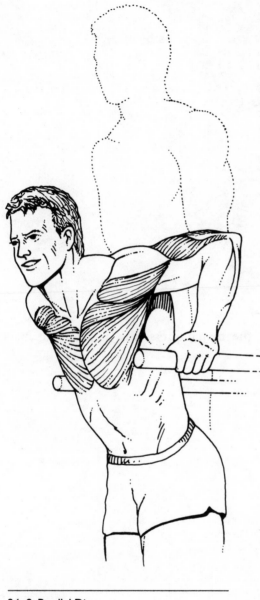

24–8. Parallel Dip

Parallel dip. Dips work the way the pectorals were designed. To hit the pectorals, lean forward into the bars, but beware if you have a bad shoulder.

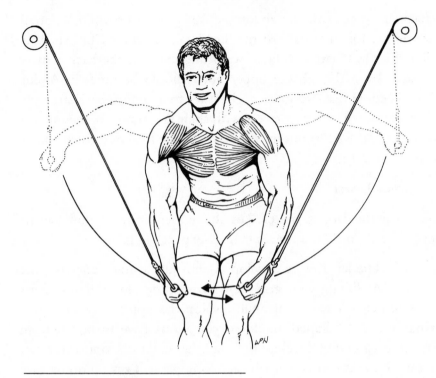

24–9. Bent-Forward Cable Crossover

Bent-forward cable crossover. A great way to get at your lower and inner pecs. Most of the development is in the squeeze at the end.

BACK

The back is a huge, largely ignored area that can provide an enormous opportunity for building new, young muscle. When you run out of development with the obvious arm and chest muscles, this is the fertile new ground to plow. Many men prefer training only body parts they can see in the mirror, but be warned that a poorly trained back leaves a weak link for most sports, since the back is the key connection between the strength of the lower-body and upper-body performance. The power generated by the lower body must be transferred to the upper body for many athletic activities: baseball swings, tennis serves, and driving in golf.

Back muscles assist the abdominal muscles in providing support and stability for the torso. At the Steadman Hawkins Clinic in Vail, Colorado, Dr. Charles Dillman was stunned to see the back activity in skiers. Even though the upper body should be quiet in Alpine skiing, keeping it stable and upright takes tremendous back strength. When you see pictures of racers with their skis almost perpendicular to the snow, the latissimus muscles take a huge load of the centrifugal force in the turn.

Latissimus Dorsi

These are the largest muscles of the upper body. If you haven't worked hard on these muscles before, expect big gains.

Chin-up. The lats can be developed with just a single exercise, the chin-up. Modifying your grip allows you to develop different parts of the muscle. A wide grip will develop the upper and outer lats, giving you that "draped" look, so you won't have to buy it from Armani. A close grip develops the lower lats and the serratus anterior, the muscles that make your rib cage look great. Plan on doing fifty chin-ups at a sitting. You may eke out only three or four per set, but still try to force your way through to a total of fifty. Remember, even very strong athletes don't punch out much more than eighteen at a time. This is a super core exercise that develops the lats and biceps, but it's an exercise that many men can't perform. That's where technology can make a big difference.

I had never been able to do many chin-ups until I began writing this book. I started with a Cybex chinning machine that allows you to rest some of your body weight by standing on a bar at the base of the machine. You can subtract anywhere from sixteen to over a hundred pounds from your body weight. That makes chins possible for virtually any man. I started chins with the machine supporting eighty pounds and ended up doing twelve or more chins per set with the machine supporting none of my weight. The beauty of these machines is they allow men who could never do any chins to begin immediately with great form and steady progress.

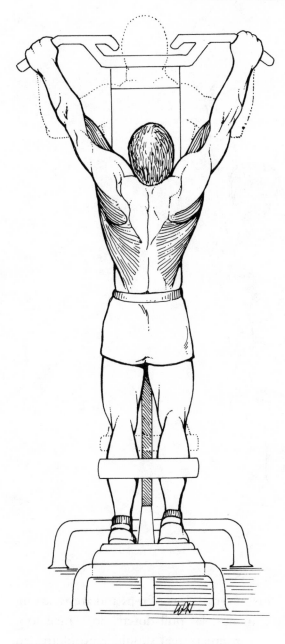

24–10. Chin-up

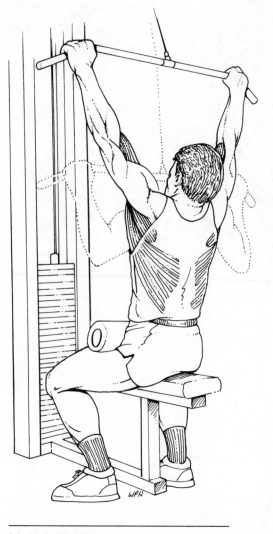

24–11. Lat Pull-down

Lat pull-down. If you want lots of sets of lots of reps and aren't strong enough to get them with chin-ups, lat pull-downs do a nice job. Behind-the-neck pull-downs can create real shoulder problems, so keep them in front if you have a bad shoulder or start to get shoulder pain. If you're just starting to train for the first time, lat pull-downs are great preparation for chin-ups.

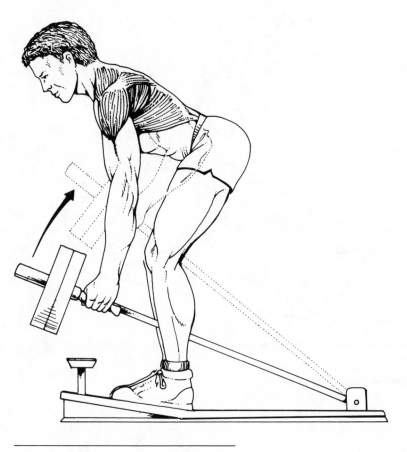

24–12. T-Bar Row

T-bar row. This is a wonderful exercise that feels like you're getting at the whole back, although the development is mostly upper lats. Be sure to push your shoulders all the way back at the end of the lift.

Decline seated cable row. I like these cable rows as a great way of getting at the lower lats. I use the weight to stretch my lower back at the end of each rep by letting it pull at my back for several seconds before the next rep. My favorite is the decline seated row machine made by Cybex. It provides great stretch to the lower back and is terrific for the lower lats as well. It is the most natural way I've found to get at the lower back muscles without overstraining them.

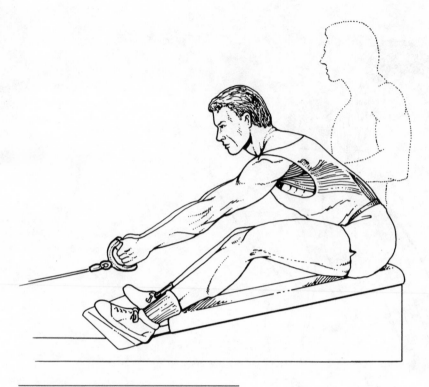

24–13. Decline Seated Cable Row

ARMS

Triceps

These muscles make up the biggest muscle mass in your arm, forming two-thirds of its bulk. If you don't train them, you'll never appear to have decent-sized arms. As a muscle with large bulk, they're a great way to build youth and easily outrank the biceps.

Triceps dip. You can't blast the triceps harder than making it lift your body weight. The trick here is to lean back into your triceps rather than forward into your pecs. If you can't perform more than four or five, try the dip machines in gyms that allow you to support some of your own weight by standing on a moving bar so you can build up

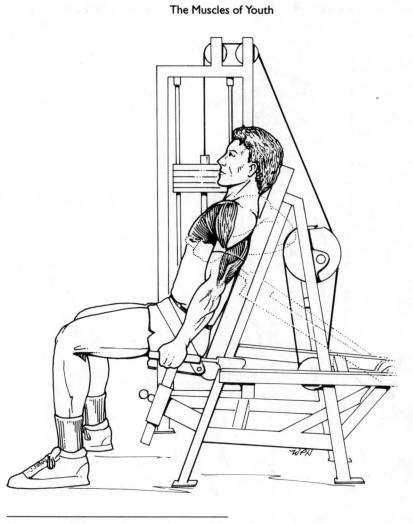

24–14. Triceps Dip

a larger volume of dips. If I'm on the road without any equipment, I'll put two chairs on either side of me, place my palms on the chair seats, and do a dip between them. Stay away from dips of any kind if you have a rotator cuff problem.

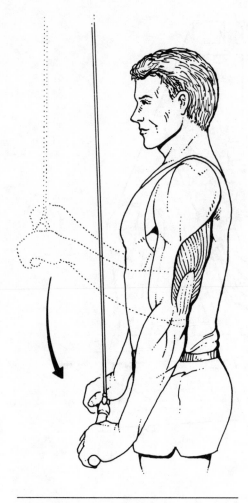

24–15. Triceps Press-down

Triceps press-down. This is a great core exercise available in virtually any gym. If you press down with your palms facing away from you, you'll work the outer triceps. By reversing your grip, so your palms face toward you, you build the inner triceps. By performing alternating sets on alternating days with the grip changed, you'll develop the classic triangular shape in your lower muscle. The elbows should remain close to the body and the exercise performed to full elbow extension.

334

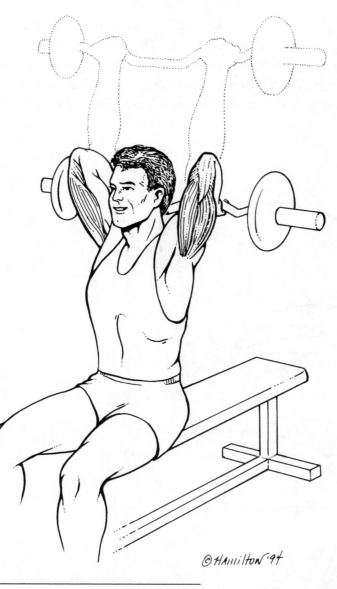

©Hamilton '94

24–16. Overhead Triceps Press

Overhead triceps press. I love this exercise because I get a great over-head shoulder flexibility drill for tennis and throwing sports. It also hits the triceps in a unique way. If I have time for only one triceps exercise, this is it.

Seated triceps press. Experts like the idea of hitting the triceps at different degrees of shoulder extension. The triceps press-down hits them at 0 degrees (elbows by your side). The overhead triceps press hits them at 180 to 200 degrees (elbows overhead). The seated triceps press hits them at 90 degrees (elbows at shoulder height in front of you).

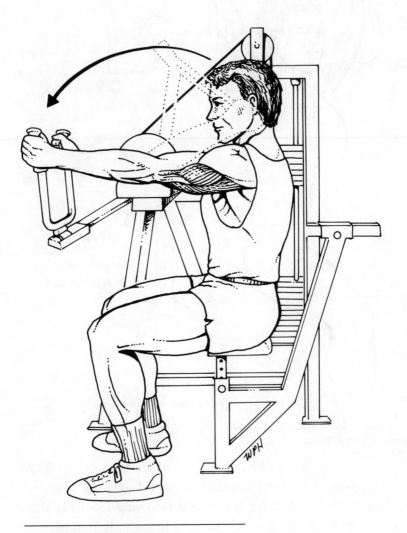

24–17. Seated Triceps Press

Biceps

Since these are core anti-frailty muscles and can develop good bulk, they're great youth-building muscles. There is a case to be made that rowing exercises for the back and pull-ups develop the biceps sufficiently, so you may not need to do separate biceps exercises if you're pressed for time. Because the biceps recover so quickly, you can use them one day for chin-ups and still be recovered adequately to use them for rows the next.

Biceps curl. This simple and universally available exercise is all you have to do for the biceps. The key is to flex your legs slightly, tighten your abdominal muscles, and practice strict form so you don't injure your back. Biceps curl machines may better isolate the biceps so you don't cheat by using your body to throw the weights up. While you can cheat the biceps curl as an advanced bodybuilder, you risk injury if you're not. If your gym has Arm Blaster bars, you can lock your elbows out of lateral play to practice strict form. Biceps machines that use cables can pretty effectively hit the biceps with little secondary muscle use. Once you've exhausted your development on the machines, try the standing barbell and preacher curl with free weights.

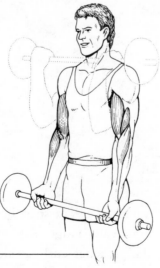

24–18. Biceps Curl

24–19A. Preacher Curl

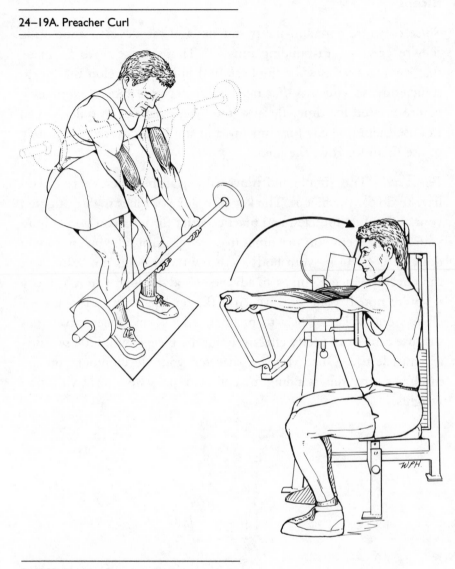

24–19B. Machine Preacher Curl

Preacher curl. I like the way this exercise stretches the biceps. It develops the muscle better in its early range of motion. If you flex your wrist during the curl, the preacher curl can develop your forearms as well.

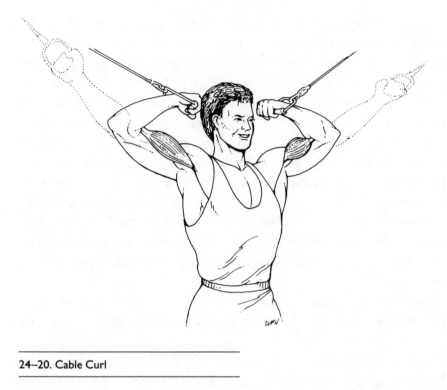

24–20. Cable Curl

Cable curl. This is a great way to hammer the biceps without the need for strong forearms. I think it delivers the most direct hit at the biceps. I use a crossover cable machine, using the upper set of cables, keeping my upper arm parallel with the cable.

LEGS AND THIGHS

Thighs and Buttocks

One weekend last winter I played in a tennis tournament against a fifty-nine-year-old named Bob O'Neil. He looked his age until he came up and leaped over the net with ease and inches to spare. I was stunned. I know few twenty-year-olds who could replicate the feat. This man demonstrated that despite his aging face, he still had the powerful, explosive leg strength that underlies excellence in every sport in this book.

339

Want to keep up with the kids? Develop strong, explosive thighs. Since as much as 60 percent of your knee strength comes from the muscles of the thighs, they are also your strongest hedge against injury. No muscles are more important in old age than those in your thighs. It may sound weird to talk about frailty when you are just thirty or forty, but look at your friends get out of a chair. How many push themselves up with their hands on their thighs? Those that do are already losing basic muscle functions. They'll blame "bad knees," but the fact is that their quadriceps muscles have just gotten too weak for their age and too weak to avoid serious injury in sports. By old age, they'll be truly frail, barely able to get up from a chair or to climb stairs. If you have parents or friends who are in their sixties or older, try to convince them at least to undertake strengthening their quads.

Both the leg press and the lunge get these muscles: quadriceps, hamstrings, gluteus maximus, or quads/hamstrings/gluts.

Leg press. No other single exercise works the muscles, tendons, and ligaments of the thighs, hips, and legs as well as the squat. You can develop the quads, hamstrings, buttocks, and even calf muscles with squats. Because squats spread the load over so many muscle groups in the upper and lower body, it is considered the number one muscle builder of all. If you could choose to do only one weight training exercise, this should be it. You're also uniquely enhancing the strength and stability of the knee joint. Mickey Levinson, P.T., clinical director of the Sportsmedicine Research and Performance Center at the Hospital for Special Surgery in New York, says, "By using the muscles on the back and the front of the thigh, you are enhancing the stability of the joint. It's a way to prevent injury and create stability."

I'm very careful not to injure my knees or back with squats. I had used a standing squat machine but found it really put undue stress on my back. What I like best is the leg press machine. By getting your feet forward to the far edge of the platform, you take the maximum amount of stress away from the knees. I use a lower weight for full

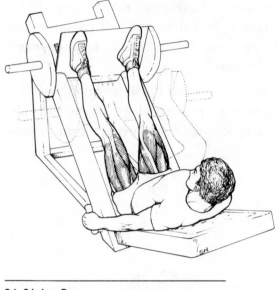

24–21. Leg Press

squats to avoid adding too much stress to the knees. The advantage of doing full squats is that you use much more hamstring and buttocks. The leg press machine can give you a huge margin of safety, so you don't strain your knees or back.

Since squats are so demanding, you should consider doing them before a long aerobic workout rather than after. You'll pump more iron that way. Although researchers are now charging that the original study that claimed squats are bad for the knees was poorly done, I still believe in protecting the knees by using heavy weights only for half squats. When you squat down, you should be able to see your toes. If you're bringing your knees forward, you're not doing it right. Be very careful not to get your knees in front of your toes or to let your knees drift outside the straight line between your hip and toes. Both can put harmful pressure on the knees. So can bouncing at the lowest point in the squat. Those three maneuvers account for most of the injuries that have given squats an unjustifiably bad name. I don't do either leg extensions or curls because the squats develop the same muscles and prepare them better for sports.

Although squats are great for the hamstrings, they do need to be stretched afterward since very tight hamstrings will compress the knees, worsening anterior knee pain. Squats are not recommended for men with lower-back problems.

Lunge. Once you can press two and a half times your body weight, you may consider lunges to improve explosive leg strength, but only if you have great knees. Use light weights and perfect form to prevent injuries.

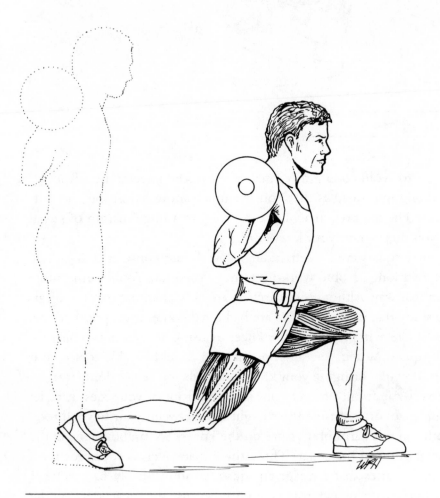

24–22. Lunge

Physical therapists and coaches are now learning that only "closed-chain" exercises provide the strength that translates to sports. Closed-chain means that there is real-life ground contact, so that all the muscles in the chain are linked to real-life movements. Mickey Levinson says, "Very often people who tend to have problems with their kneecap do better with the closed-chain exercises. Leg extensions place tremendous sheering forces on the knee if you go to full extension and can make a bad knee worse." Mickey has this warning: "More and more we're tending to rehab people without using the knee extension. Although it is the best way to isolate the quad muscle, it's also the best way to irritate the kneecap. If you have someone with an unstable knee, when they kick out during a knee extension, it will make their tibia, their shinbone, slide forward in relation to their thighbone. This of course creates a lot of problems."

ABDOMINALS

The abdominals are the most powerful stabilizing muscles of the back, making them important anti-frailty muscles and critical for any sport linking the power of the upper and lower body. You can develop bulk in the abdominal muscles, but not with traditional calisthenics. The abdominal crunch machine and the Rotary Torso get these muscles: rectus abdominus/obliques.

Abdominal crunch. I'm a big fan of abdominal machines. They are quick, efficient, and painless. I find crunches, sit-ups, leg raises, and most other calisthenic exercises uncomfortable and not all that effective. I use a Cybex upper abdominal machine in the gym. I lift all fourteen plates, so I'm getting a real power workout, developing good mass with a very nice feel to the exercise. Cybex also makes a nice rotary machine for the abdominals called the Rotary Torso. The biggest breakthrough is the AB Flexor, a machine for the lower abdominals made by FLEX Equipment, Inc., of Corona, California. Again, it's so much more mechanically efficient and correct than crunches or leg raises that it's a real pleasure to use.

343

The abdominals, like the biceps, recover very quickly and can be worked at least three times a week.

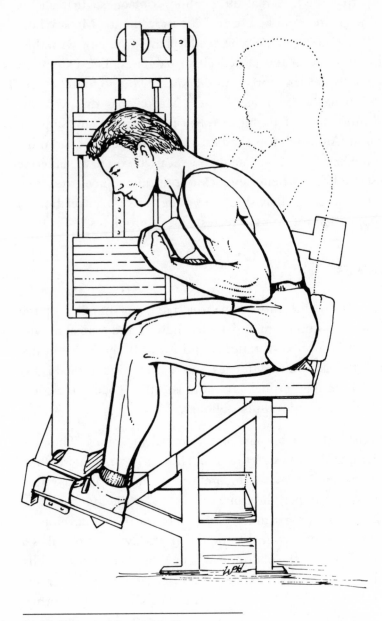

24–23. Abdominal Crunch Machine

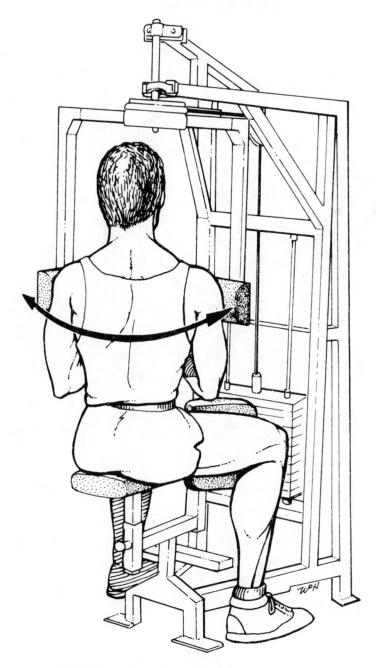

24–24. Rotary Torso

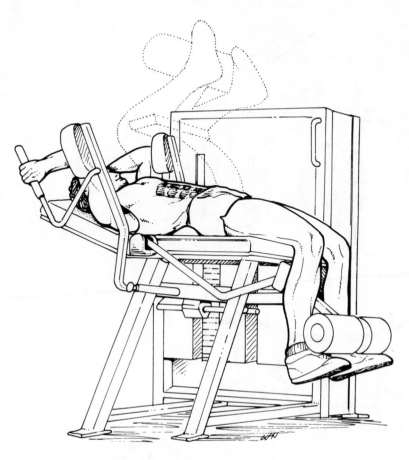

24–25. AB Flexor Machine

Chapter 25

Choosing a Routine

THE HEADLINES FROM MUSCLE AND FITNESS MAGAZINES TRUMPET NEW surefire methods every month to "blast your pecs" or develop "killer biceps." None of these programs contain any remarkably new ideas. What works best is well understood by researchers. The programs will work because the muscle is getting a fresh new stimulus, but no one program has any more magic than another. The best advice is to pick a program that has solid fundamentals and lots of diversity.

> Conventional Wisdom:
> *There's a secret key to success.*
> New Paradigm:
> *Every program works at the right time in your development.*

THE BASICS

If you've never trained before, you'll quickly discover that "reps" and "sets" are the basic language of weight training. A "rep" is one complete cycle of lifting and lowering a weight. A "set" is the number of times the weight is lifted and lowered before fatigue makes it impossible to lift the weight one last time. The number of repetitions in a set is determined by the weight you choose. The lighter the weight, the more repetitions you can perform.

In theory, you need to test yourself to determine what the greatest weight you can lift just once is. In practice, there are very few non-professional weight lifters who have the technique or strength to make this a very meaningful test. The most practical way of getting a handle on an exercise is to determine how many repetitions you can perform with a given weight. When you get into the range of eight to twelve repetitions, you're in the training zone. If you have to struggle so hard that you can't practice good form, you've got too much weight. The good news is that you needn't have exceptional strength, nor must you be able to handle very heavy loads to get great results. This eight-to-twelve range allows you to do enough repetitions that you'll get a great training effect. Just as a marathoner piles up hundreds of miles to get a training effect, a bodybuilder wants to pile up a big volume of repetitions.

In order to hit the muscle hard enough often enough, repetitions are divided up into multiple sets. Training to failure at the end of each set is what counts most. This simply means that you can't lift the weight again after your last repetition.

Three is pretty much the minimum number of sets. I usually go for four if I have the time. If I really have a sticking point with a muscle where I'm showing no improvement, I'll do six sets of one exercise. Although some advanced bodybuilders advocate breath holding to increase the weight they can lift, extremely high blood pressures may result. Normal is 120/80. Researchers have observed pressure higher than 400/300!

The first set is conventionally a warm-up set with twelve to fifteen repetitions so that the muscle isn't injured. Here's what the different numbers of reps do for you, assuming each set is to failure.

Goal	Repetitions
Pure strength	2–5
Bulk	8–12
Warm-up	12–15
Endurance	15+

The higher the intensity the more recovery you need. After a single rep to maximum power, you need several minutes to be able to lift that single rep again. That's because the energy system for maximum exertion takes that long to recover. At low intensities, you need almost no recovery. Since you want to make lots of lactic acid as a training stimulus, shorter rest periods or supersets (see below) are a great way to build lots of lactic acid for intermediate loads.

You could invent dozens of different ways of doing sets, and the experts have. The kinds of sets you will do form the core of any good training program. Here's what works.

Increasing Weight

Proponents of increasing the weight with each set say that the muscle "remembers" the last weight it lifted and this should be the heaviest. After a warm-up of ten to twelve reps, you might try sets of eight to ten, six to eight, and four to six reps.

Decreasing Weight

A review of the research shows that decreasing weight with each set may produce slightly better results than increasing the weight with each set. After a warm-up of ten to twelve repetitions, you might try the following sets: three to five, six to eight, and eight to ten reps to failure. Go for a good pump in the last set by lowering the weight and increasing the rep.

Supersets

The superset typically works opposing muscle groups in alternating sets. Here's an example. Do twelve biceps curls followed immediately by twelve triceps press-downs. Repeat the cycle two or three more times. By cutting out the rest period, you're saving as much as eight minutes over the time it would take to work each muscle individually. I can get my heart rate into the 140s and keep it there. I'm convinced this is the nineties version of circuit training. A series of supersets provides a great aerobic workout and no compromise on weight training. Other examples of supersets:

- Overhead presses and lat pull-downs.
- Chin-ups and triceps dips.

The only downside of supersets is that you've got to be pretty fit. I waited until my third month of weight training to try them.

The American College of Sports Medicine advocates weight training twice a week at a minimum, three times a week for significant strength increases. Research shows that four times a week is even better.

"Hit the biggest muscles first while they're fresh" has been the battle cry of American bodybuilding for decades. Since those are the most powerful anti-aging muscles, that still makes sense. There's no proof that any other system works better. You should be aware that the old Eastern Bloc sports machines tried exhausting the small muscles first and then moving up to the larger muscles. Unless you're a highly experienced bodybuilder, you probably won't like this small-to-large scheme.

Progression

The first few months of bodybuilding are the best you'll ever have. You'll make big gains in strength during the first month. Then you'll begin to see harder, firmer muscle and finally bigger muscle. You almost can't go wrong in choosing a method to train by. But just as you're feeling terrific and certain you'll go on to build bigger and firmer and better muscles . . . it all stops. You may even slide backward on the weights you can lift. It's called a plateau and every bodybuilder from Arnold Schwarzenegger to Sylvester Stallone has hit it. The best way to beat staleness is through advanced planning to outsmart the muscle. That's done by varying the intensity of your workout in cycles that progress from light to moderate to heavy. The simplest method of periodizing is to change at the beginning of every month. Here's how:

Month	Reps	Sets
January	10–12	4–5
February	6–8	3–5
March	4–6	3–5

Then repeat the same cycle for April, May, and June, and so on.

The prevailing wisdom from the 1970s was that it took seventy-two hours for a muscle to recover. In truth, different muscles vary in their ability to recover. For instance, the biceps, triceps, and abdominal muscles recover very quickly, whereas the lower-back muscles can take a week. I like to give chest, back, and legs a long recovery. Since recovery slows as you age, many men are now working major muscle groups once a week. I will go through training cycles where I train one body part a day for five days. That gives me incredible recovery, so I can hit the muscles hard with lots of sets from many different angles. The best indication that your muscles haven't recovered is that they are still sore. The second best is that you can't lift as much.

Speed

Coaches say that you want to train muscle near the speed at which it will be used. For general strength training, an intermediate speed gives you increases in strength above and below that speed. Closer to your sport season, you may want to increase the speed to meet that of the actual sport. The most interesting new research shows that high-speed training increases the elasticity of the muscle. Since you lose elasticity with aging, this is a critical breakthrough. A load of 30 percent of maximum produces the greatest elasticity. Performance is increased more by high-speed training than low-speed training, in part because you must improve coordination at high speed to be able to use it. The more sport-specific and fast the training, the more it will transfer to your sport. This needs to be added on top of an extremely powerful base of lower-speed training, since high-speed training runs a greater risk of tendonitis or actual muscle tears. For instance, you won't want to do high-speed leg training until you can squat with at least twice your weight. Although not sport-specific, isokinetic machines allow very high speed training in a very safe environment. Rather than setting a weight to lift, isokinetic machines allow you to choose a fixed speed at which to train. The only quibble exercise physiologists have is that this is not a closed-chain exercise. That is, there is no ground contact and so its usefulness in sport is less than those exercises that allow contact from the ground up. Training at an intermediate speed also increases power at faster speeds and is a safe alternative.

THE ROUTINES

Phase I

Joint Stabilization. In this fundamental first phase, your muscles, tendons, and ligaments become strong enough to withstand the forces required by weight training and stabilize your joints to prevent injury. This essential first step creates the levers of power needed to lift heavier weights. Ed Irace, C.P.T., owner of SPARTA (Sports Performance and Resistance Training Arena) in New York, says, "The stabilization phase is for the beginner who wants to take on strength conditioning seriously. He's going to need this step to build a good strong foundation on which to work and really make gains."

In the stabilization program, machines are suggested instead of free weights. Since you can move only within the limits the machine allows, you are being taught the appropriate range of motion and muscle use. Each exercise is performed every day you train, which should be three days a week. Do three to five sets of eight to twelve reps each. The stabilization program is only for those men who don't lift at all. After six to eight weeks, you're ready for phase two.

Phase I Exercises: Days 1, 3, and 5

- Chest
  Chest press
  Fly
- Back

Seated lat pull-down with wide bar
Decline seated cable row
- **Shoulders**
Overhead press
Lateral raise
- **Biceps**
Preacher curl
Overhead triceps press
- **Legs**
Leg press
- **Abdominals**
Abdominal crunch machine

Phase 2: Building Mass

With strong ligaments and tendons, good form, and joints hardened against injury, you're now ready to really build muscle. The primary difference between phase one and phase two is the increase from one exercise per body part to three, four, or five. This provides the maximum stimulus to the muscle and is the biggest single secret in successful bodybuilding. The second difference is that you don't work every muscle group every day. The 48- to 72-hour recovery period for the major muscle groups allows you to really attack the weights with fresh muscles. You may continue using machines in phase two as long as you continue to make progress. But let's say your bench press gets stuck at one setting or your shoulders are beginning to get sore. That's the signal to move to free weights. You'll then experience another cycle of mass building. I've tried every variation and settled on this schedule:

Days 1 and 3: pectorals, shoulders, leg extensions, lunges.
Days 2 and 4: back, triceps, biceps, abdomen.

These need not be done over four consecutive days. In fact a longer interval allows better recovery. For instance, you might consider Monday, Wednesday, Thursday, and Saturday for days 1, 2, 3, and 4.

If you're pressed for time, stop at three exercises per body part. Do three to five sets. On day 1, I like to hit the pecs first with fresh triceps to get maximum push. On day 2, I'll work the back first with fresh biceps. Each month vary the number of repetitions as suggested above in the *Progression* section.

Phase 2 Exercises: Days I and 3

- Pecs
  Bench press
  Incline press
  Fly
  Bent-forward cable crossover
  Parallel dip
- Shoulders
  Upright row
  Overhead press
  Lateral raise
  Dumbbell shrug
- Legs
  Leg press
  Lunge

Days 2 and 4

- Back
  Chin-up
  Decline seated cable row
  T-bar row
- Triceps
  Overhead triceps press
  Triceps press-down
  Seated triceps press
  Triceps dip
- Biceps
  Biceps curl
  Cable curl

    Machine preacher curl
    Seated dumbbell curl
- **Abdominals**
    Abdominal crunch
    Rotary torso
    AB flexor

Phase two can take six months to several years to attain and is all you'll ever need for the purposes of this book.

Phase 3

High-Performance Maintenance. This program hits every body part heavily but just once a week, allowing each body part up to a whole week to recover. Since many muscles never get a chance to recover fully if they're hammered too often, this program is rapidly gaining favor. Training each body part on just one day a week is hard to adjust to psychologically because it feels that it's just not enough, but consider that even Mr. Olympia trains one body part per week in four forty-five-minute sessions. This is a great maintenance program if you are in an active sports season where the last thing you need is sore muscles. You'll be amazed just how hard you can hammer muscles when they're as fresh as they are in this phase. It's also a great respite if you're sore, tired, stale, or just plain sick of phase two. Since total training time per day is less than twenty minutes, all that's required is easy access to a gym.

Phase 3 Exercises:

    Day 1: back.
    Day 2: shoulders, abdominals.
    Day 3: pecs, legs.
    Day 4: biceps, abdominals.
    Day 5: triceps, legs.

I like this program because I'm never sore and can always pump each muscle group for maximum burn. I usually do four sets of four exercises per body part. If I'm really having trouble with a body part, say the pecs, then I'll do six sets of each exercise. Champion body-builders might do as many as eighteen sets to really push muscular development. You'll notice that squats and abdominals are repeated because of their faster recovery times. All upper-body muscles are worked just once. Since this is a once–a–week–per–body–part program, you should do lots of sets of lots of exercises to maximally pump and exhaust the muscle. If you want to cut the time commitment, combine days 4 and 5.

Do three to five sets. Each month vary the number of repetitions as suggested above in the *Progression* section.

Day I

- **Back**
  Chin-up
  Incline row
  Decline seated cable row
  T-bar row

Day 2

- **Shoulders**
  Overhead press
  Lateral raise
  Upright row
  Dumbbell shrug

- **Abdominals**
  Abdominal crunch machine
  AB flexor
  Rotary torso

Day 3

- **Pecs**
  Bench press
  Incline press
  Fly
  Bent-forward cable crossover
  Triceps press-down

- **Legs**
  Leg press
  Lunge

Day 4

- **Biceps**
  Biceps curl
  Preacher curl
  Cable curl

- **Abdominals**
  Abdominal crunch machine
  AB flexor
  Rotary torso

Day 5

- **Triceps**
  Triceps dip
  Triceps press-down
  Overhead triceps press

- **Legs**
  Leg press
  Lunge

Phase 4

Time-Saving Maintenance. Most men in the peak years of their careers have little time to exercise. The super-efficiency phase four allows you to maintain and even build muscles in less than an hour a week. How?

Supersets. The biggest time loss in weight training is the rest period between sets. Supersets are a terrific way to drop those rest periods. The supersets I like best match opposing groups of muscles. For instance, you may do a set of biceps curls followed by a set of triceps pull-downs. While you exercise the biceps, the triceps are resting. They will get as much rest as they would if you were just doing repetitions of triceps pull-downs with thirty seconds between sets. The trick is getting the proper machines or weights close enough together to make supersets feasible. At my gym they have one station that incorporates a lat pull-down with a bench press. I do eight repetitions of latissimus, then eight bench presses. I repeat the cycle four times. That gives me eight sets with no rest. The whole exercise takes four minutes, and I've worked out two of the biggest muscle groups. Supersets also tax the cardiovascular system, so I get a good aerobic workout as well. By doing supersets, you can perform twenty-four repetitions for twelve different muscle groups in as little as twenty minutes. If you work out only twice a week, you've got a total forty-minute investment in weight training.

Major compound exercises. You can build up lots of power and strength with just a few exercises. In fact just three exercises can hit each one of the major muscle groups. Here's how:

> *Leg press:* quads, spinal erectors, gluteus maximus, hamstrings.
> *Bench press:* pectorals, anterior deltoid, triceps.
> *Clean pull or "power clean":* quads, lats, traps, deltoids, forearm, spinal erectors.

Although exercises that isolate a single muscle may give you more definition of that muscle, compound exercises give you maximum strength and the most direct translation to sport. You may develop tremendous quad definition by exercising on a leg extension machine, but if you had done squats instead, you'd have much more power that you could use in skiing, tennis, climbing, rollerblading, and other sports.

Like many other beginners, I didn't think compound exercises were a very sexy or high-tech way to go. Part of my resistance was the inability to do them very well. That's why building up to them through phases one and two is very important. But once you can perform these exercises well, you can keep your mass up with little time expended. If you're really on the run and have to scramble for time, try this super-efficiency workout two or three times a week.

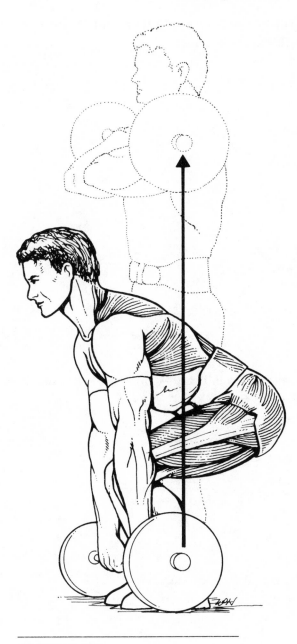

25–1. Power Clean

Do three to five sets. Each month vary the number of repetitions as suggested above in the *Progression* section.

- **Superset #1: chest**
  Fly
  Bench press
- **Superset #2: shoulders**
  Overhead press
  Upright row
- **Superset #3: back**
  Chin-up
  Decline seated cable row
- **Superset #4: abdomen, legs**
  Abdominal crunch machine
  Leg press
- **Superset #5: arms**
  Triceps dip
  Biceps curl

(If you're incredibly pressed for time, drop #5 since the other supersets will cover your biceps and triceps.)

Chapter 26

Building Elastic Muscle

ALBERTO TOMBA, THE MOST POWERFUL SKIER IN HISTORY, LEARNED quickly that all the strength in the world gained from weight training did him little good on the slalom hill until he became flexible enough to move quickly and explosively. As they near thirty and beyond, most athletes realize they can achieve the strength, power, and endurance of a teenager, but not the flexibility. I was tempted not to write a stretching chapter for this book at all, because I couldn't find a program that really worked. I never stretched until I found the program I describe here, because, like many men, I never got much out of stretching. I still see men every day in my gym sitting on the floor, legs stretched out, trying to push their heads to their knees. They strain to increase their stretch by holding out as long as they can, hoping they'll be able to hold a "static" stretch for at least fifteen seconds. What men don't know is that static stretching is on the way out. Aaron Mattes, a kinesiologist in Sarasota, Florida, states that it's potentially causing you a lot more damage and gaining you a lot less flexibility than you think.

The next generation has arrived, and it's called Active Isolated Stretching. Although scientists have been researching this technique for over twenty-five years and Olympians have been employing it for about eight years, AI stretching has only recently been brought to the public's attention, mostly by the efforts of Jim and Phil Wharton. This father-and-son team, educated by pioneer Aaron Mattes, work out of their clinic, Maximum Performance International, in New York City. "This is the first form of stretching that respects how the body works," says Jim Wharton. I thought my hips were shot until Jim took me through the hip flexion exercises. To my delight, he showed that my hips were locked and could easily be unchained with AI stretching.

"We do activity day in and day out that is very muscle-specific, so we lose our elasticity in those muscles that we don't use. We even lose elasticity in the muscles we do use because we do not take those movements through a full range of motion," says Jim Wharton. With AI stretching, you can dramatically increase your flexibility in a number of days. I was astounded to realize increases of 40 degrees in my hip range of motion.

Out of the many individuals the Whartons have trained, thirty-three are Olympians, eleven of whom have medaled. After working with Dennis Mitchell, the 1992 bronze medalist in the 100-meter dash, for just a year, his time dropped from 10.03 seconds to 9.91. According to Jim Wharton, with AI stretching, vertical jumping has improved, and says Phil Wharton, "In specific athletes, we've gotten an extra foot on the long jump and triple jump." Phil and Jim Wharton have also trained the therapists working with Alberto Tomba. Deep-muscle stretching has allowed Tomba to transform incredible strength into explosive power by making it elastic and springy rather than stiff and slow. A phenomenal example is Jack Pierce, the 1992 silver medalist in the 110-meter hurdles. "Jack came to us in 1991 with a doctors-diagnosed torn hamstring. He was on crutches and hadn't run for two weeks. In less than eleven days, we got him back and ready to compete and he won." Today he still practices AI stretching. The Whartons have worked with four major universities, all of which have reduced injuries and increased performance.

"Within one year," Phil Wharton says, "the Michigan women's track team went from eighth in the conference with sixty percent injuries to first in the conference with nearly zero percent injuries."

Most men play a variety of sports with their hips almost locked up. They mistake this condition for aging and simply slow down and limit their movements. AI stretching almost miraculously unlocks your hips so that you have the free-floating pelvis of a child. Much of that is by unbinding the connective tissue (fascia) that so tightly constricts movement with age.

AI stretching will reduce your workload in most sports by removing tightness so you can swing your limbs more freely. It transports oxygen to sore muscles and quickly removes toxins from muscles, so recovery is faster. And AI stretching is an alternative to what Wharton calls the "massage dependency loop." Says Jim Wharton, "So many athletes use massage in order to maintain muscle elasticity and to flush out toxins from exercise. AI stretching is deeper than massage because we're involving and activating the muscle fibers while we're stretching. Even deep tissue massage is still a passive activity." I still advocate massage, but it's too expensive to be used on an everyday basis, whereas AI stretching is free.

AI stretching isolates muscles in novel and well-thought-out ways. Even if you're a veteran stretcher, you'll be struck by how specifically you stretch exactly where you need it the most. Explains Jim Wharton, "Isolated stretching is just that, isolated. It's critical to stretch one muscle at a time. That's what's wrong with the guy in the gym on the floor, trying to touch his knee with his head. He's trying to stretch his back and his hamstrings at the same time. If you do that, you're literally pitting one muscle group against the other making you more prone to injury."

In AI stretching, contracting muscles are the main force that causes the opposing muscle to elongate or stretch. As one muscle works, the opposite, the antagonist, relaxes. For instance, the hamstring is used to stretch the quadriceps. Each stretch position is held only to the point of mild discomfort, roughly two seconds. Jim Wharton explains: "If you hold for a longer period of time, a signal comes in from the brain and says, 'Wait a minute. I have to lock up that muscle to protect it from overstretching.' It's an automatic defense mechanism." Put simply, you will be trying to stretch a tight muscle and can injure or irritate it. It will keep the muscle tight. That's why so many men say they stretch and stretch and stretch, but don't get any more flexible. It's because they're not really creating a vibrant, elastic muscle. "The way to create that flexibility is to hold for two seconds only," says Jim Wharton.

After holding the stretch for two seconds, you return to your starting point, relax, and repeat this same movement eight to ten times, each time easing more and more into the movement. In some of the movements you wrap a rope around your foot and pull gently for increased leverage. "The muscles work all the way through the movement. At the end of the movement, the rope is pulled and assists the stretch so that each time, you go a little further," Jim Wharton says.

AI stretching is a monitoring system for your flexibility, balance, and strength. "Stretching," says Jim Wharton, "is just the tip of what we do. By stretching one muscle at a time, it allows you to really, specifically feel whether or not it's tight, and if it's continually tight, you become aware that either it's being overworked or it's compensating for another muscle group that's either weak or inflexible. So it's a monitoring system that allows you to bring your flexibility and your strength into balance."

GENERAL DIRECTIONS FOR AI STRETCHING

Lift Through the Entire Range of Motion

"You have to keep reminding people that the working muscle continues to work through the full range of motion. At the end of the stretch, you assist with the rope as you continue to work the muscle," says Jim Wharton.

Increase the Range of Motion with Each Repetition

The key is to return to the starting position after each repetition and repeat, attempting to gently increase your range of motion with each repetition.

Maintain the Stretch for Only Two Seconds

A lot of men want to stay in the stretch because it feels good. But the short duration of the stretch and the ten repetitions that follow are the foundation of the program.

Breathe Properly

Exhale as you stretch, inhale as the body part returns to the starting position. "Breathing is a big part of AI stretching. You must always exhale when you work. That's the time when you are bringing the blood and the new oxygen to the isolated area," says Jim Wharton. You'll notice a warm, satisfying feeling in the area you've just finished stretching as the blood rushes in.

Relax

Let the other parts of your body relax. "Some people tense up their shoulders and neck as they stretch their legs. It's important to stay relaxed," says Jim Wharton.

Of the dozens of AI stretches, the following program concentrates on the key youth-building movements. If you want to shorten this program even further, concentrate only on those stretches where you notice the greatest burn. That's where you'll benefit the most. For each exercise perform ten repetitions. Hold each repetition for two seconds. Lie down, if you'll be using more than one muscle, to prevent injury. This series begins with exercises to unlock the hip. That eases strain on the lower back and gives you the hip mobility of a kid. You should stretch every day, but even twice a week is highly effective.

HIPS AND TRUNK

Sports scientists and leading-edge coaches are beginning to realize that the hips, as the body's center of gravity, are critical to a wide range of sports. It's the hips that provide the most dynamic power in

Alpine skiing, speed skating, ice hockey, cross-country skiing, tennis, golf, and even baseball. Few athletes devote much time to training the hips, but strong, flexible hip muscles allow you to coil, power, and blast into a ski turn, tennis stroke, or golf shot.

1. **Pelvic Tilt** (knee to chest)
   Muscles stretched: low back and outer buttocks
   Muscles contracting: hip flexor and abdominal muscles

   Lie on your back with both legs flat on the ground. Keep the left leg straight on the floor. Contract the hip flexor and abdominal muscles to lift the right thigh toward your chest. Pull your thigh into your chest by continuing to contract your hip flexors and abdominal muscles. Assist with both hands behind the right thigh only as you near the chest to increase the range of motion. Hold for two seconds and release. Allow your lower right leg to fall into a naturally relaxed position as you draw your thigh to your chest. Do ten reps. Repeat with the left leg.

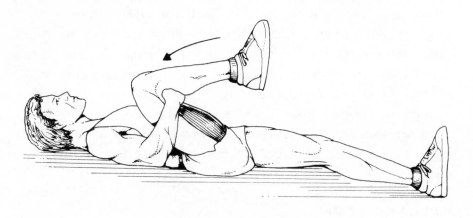

26–1. Pelvic Tilt

366

2. **Pelvic Tilt II** (double knee to chest)
   Muscles stretched: low back and outer buttocks
   Muscles contracting: hip flexor and abdominal muscles

   Lie on your back. Bring both knees to your chest, allowing your lower legs to fall into a naturally relaxed position. As your legs near the chest, pull even closer with both hands on the backs of your thighs. Hold for two seconds and release. Extend your legs until they are flat on the floor after each repetition. Do ten reps.

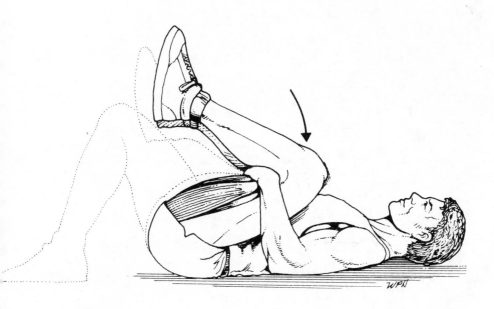

26–2. Pelvic Tilt II

3. Hamstring — Bent Knee

Muscles stretched: lower hamstring
Muscles contracting: quadriceps muscles

Lie on your back. Keep your left foot flat on the floor with the left knee bent at about 90 degrees. Pull your right thigh as close to your chest as possible by pulling it toward you with a rope wrapped around the arch of your right foot. Keep your right lower leg parallel to the ground. Hold the rope with your right hand. Contract the right quadriceps muscles to extend the right leg to a lock-out position. You'll feel a nice clean pull through your hamstrings. Hold for two seconds and release. Do ten reps. Repeat with the left leg.

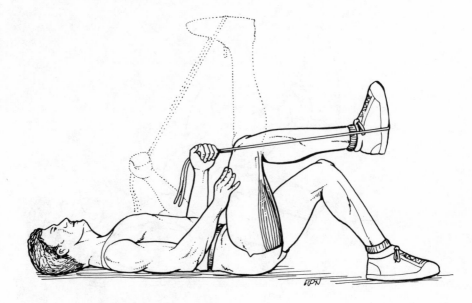

26–3. Hamstring — Bent Knee

4. Hamstring — Straight Leg

Muscles stretched: hamstring muscles
Muscles contracting: quadriceps and hip flexor muscles

Lie on your back. Keep the left foot flat on the floor with the left knee bent at a right angle. Wrap your rope around the arch of the right foot with the right leg fully extended on the floor and the right knee locked. Contract the right quadriceps and hip flexor muscles to pull the right leg up toward the head, leaving the knee locked. Use your hands on the rope to give gentle assistance at the end of the movement. Hold for two seconds and release. Do ten reps. Repeat with the left leg.

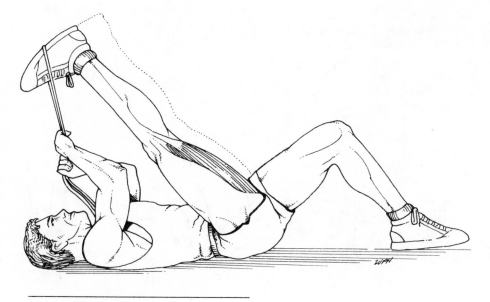

26–4. Hamstring — Straight Leg

5. **Hip Adductor**

Muscles stretched: inner thigh and groin
Muscles contracting: hip and thigh muscle group, middle buttocks

Lie on your back with both legs flat on the floor. Wrap a rope around the arch of your right foot. Point the toes of your right foot toward the midline of your left leg. Move the right leg away from the left leg with your right leg just clearing the floor. Gently assist with the rope to move your right leg as far from your left leg as possible. Hold for two seconds and release. Do ten reps. Repeat with the left leg.

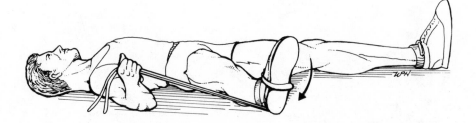

26–5. Hip Adductor

6. Hip Abductor

Muscles stretched: outer thigh and hip; middle buttocks

Muscles contracting: adductor muscle group

Lie on your back. Extend both legs. Place the rope around the arch of your right leg. Point the toes of your right foot away from your left foot, keeping your right knee locked. With your right leg low to the ground, move it across your left leg and then as far as you can to the left by gently assisting with the rope. Hold for two seconds and release. Do ten reps. Repeat with the left leg.

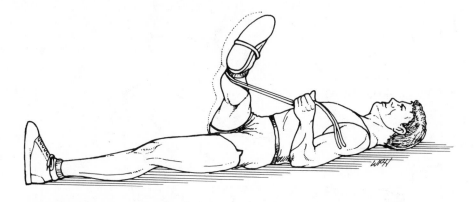

26–6. Hip Abductor

7. Quadriceps

Muscles stretched: front of thigh

Muscles contracting: abdominal muscles, outer buttocks, and hamstrings

Lie on your left side. Bring both knees toward your chest so you are in a fetal position. Stabilize your left knee by holding it with your left hand. Grab your right ankle with your right hand. Contract your abdominal muscles to prevent your pelvis from tilting. Contract your gluteal muscles and hamstrings to bring your right thigh backward. Gently pull your right heel go-

ing toward your butt with your right hand. Hold for two seconds and release. Do ten reps. Repeat with the left leg.

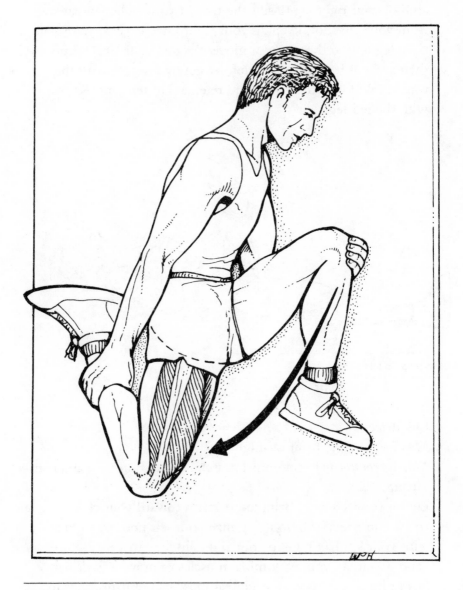

26–7. Quadriceps

8. **Reverse Trunk:** modified diagonal knee to shoulder
   Muscles stretched: lateral hip and buttock
   Muscles contracting: abdominal and hip flexor muscles
   Lie on your back. Keep your left leg flat on the floor. Rotate
   your left foot toward your right foot to stabilize your hips. Bend
   your right knee to a right angle with your right foot flat on the
   floor. Contract the hip flexor and abdominal muscles and bring
   the right knee to the left shoulder. Gently assist with the left
   hand on the right shin and the right hand on the right outer
   thigh. Hold for two seconds and release. Do ten reps. Repeat
   with the left leg.

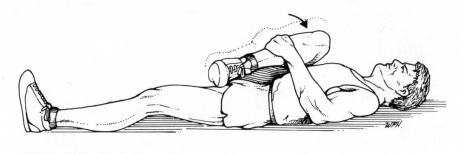

26–8. Reverse Trunk

9. **Up and Over** (piriformis)
   Muscles stretched: muscles in the lower back and hip responsible
     for rotational movements; outer buttocks, middle buttocks, and
     the piriformis, which is next to the deepest portion of the but-
     tocks
   Muscles contracting: lower abdominals, internal hip rotators, and
     hip flexors
   Lie on your back. Rotate the left foot toward the right foot.
   Wrap your rope around the arch of the right foot. Extend your
   right leg in a locked-out position and raise the leg as high as possible. Then contract your muscles to bring your leg straight
   across your body as far to the left as you can. Hold for two

seconds and release. Gently assist with the rope. Do ten reps. Repeat with the left leg.

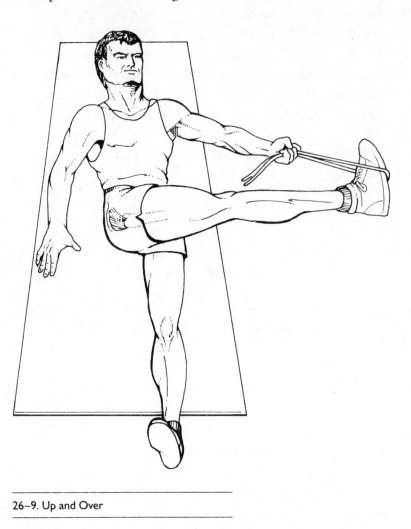

26–9. Up and Over

10. **Medial Hip Rotator** (inside hip)
    Muscles stretched: deep buttock muscles
    Muscles contracting: outer buttocks and external hip rotators
    Sit on the floor with your back straight. Place the left leg in a locked-out position straight on the floor and keep it there.

Take your right leg and bend it so that its ankle will rest on your left thigh, just an inch above your right knee. Now contract your buttocks and external hip rotators to drive your left outer knee toward the floor. Gently assist by pressing on the inner thigh with both hands. Hold for two seconds and release. Do ten reps. Repeat with the left leg.

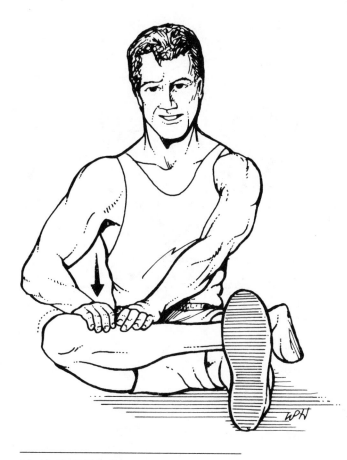

26–10. Medial Hip Rotator

11. Trunk Flexion — Bent Leg

Muscles stretched: back muscles, which extend from the base of the skull to the pelvis along the spinal column, and the muscles of the lower back

Muscles contracting: abdominal muscles

Sit on the floor with both of your knees bent at a right angle. Strongly contract your abdominal muscles as your upper body reaches down toward the floor between your knees. With your hands on your ankles, gently assist at the end of the movement. Hold for two seconds and release. Do ten reps.

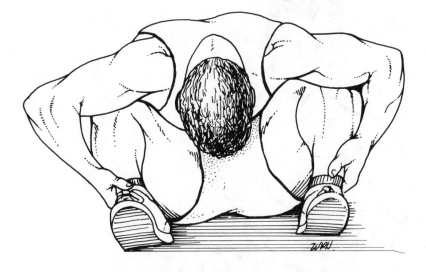

26–11. Trunk Flexion — Bent Leg

12. Middle calf (soleus)

Muscles stretched: inner calf muscle

Muscles contracting: shin muscles

Sit on the floor with the left leg relaxed on the floor. The right leg should be bent at a 90-degree angle. Place your hands on the ball of your right foot and use the shin to lift the forefoot off the floor. Do not lift the whole foot. The heel stays on the floor. Hold for two seconds and release. Do ten reps. Repeat with the left leg.

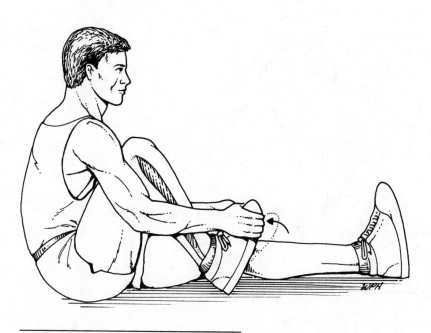

26–12. Middle Calf

13. **Outer calf** (gastrocnemius)
   Muscles stretched: outer calf muscle
   Muscles contracting: shin muscles
   Sit on the floor with both legs flat on the floor. Relax the left leg. Put the right leg straight out in front of you and lock the knee. Wrap your rope around the ball of your right foot. Use your right shin to bring your toes toward your head. In the first few repetitions, the upper body is not moving at all. As you continue to repeat the movement, you can move the up-

per trunk downward, more toward the knee. You should feel this stretch behind the knee. Hold for two seconds and release. Do ten reps. Repeat with the left leg.

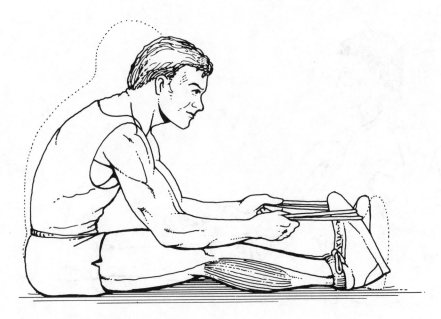

26–13. Outer Calf

14. **Trunk flexion** (side reach)
   Muscles stretched: same muscles as contracting muscles, but the opposite side
   Muscles contracting: all muscles at the side of the lower back
   Stand keeping your pelvis level. Put your hands behind your head and reach laterally to the right side as far as possible. Hold for two seconds and release. Do ten reps. Do the same with the left side.

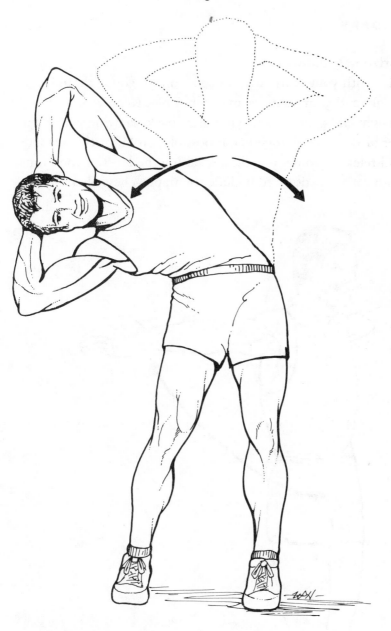

26–14. Trunk Flexion

SHOULDERS

15. Horizontal Abduction

Stand with your arms raised out in front of you at shoulder height and your palms facing each other. Keep your arms straight and gently throw your arms back, drawing your shoulder blades as close together as possible. Hold for two seconds and release. Do ten repetitions, raising the level of your arms with each repetition to include the upper-chest fibers.

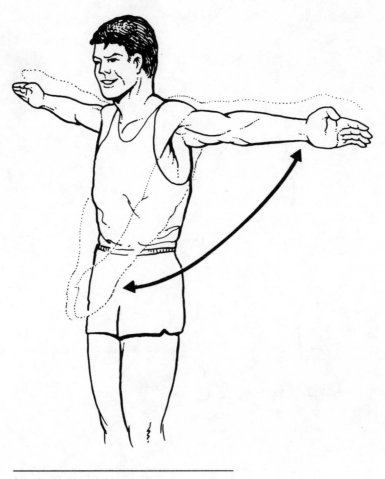

26–15. Horizontal Abduction

16. Internal Rotation

Stand with your elbows bent at a 90-degree angle, level with your shoulders, hands pointed forward with your palms facing down. Keeping your elbows level with your shoulders, rotate your forearm downward as far as possible so that your palms face behind you. Tighten the muscles in your shoulder to keep the shoulder blade from rotating. Do a slow, steady stretch at the end of the movement. Hold for two seconds and release. Repeat fifteen times. Repeat with the left arm.

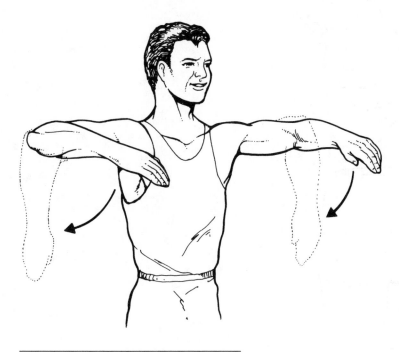

26–16. Internal Rotation

17. Horizontal Flexion

Place your right hand on your left shoulder. Walk your right hand as far down your spinal column as possible. Place your left hand on your right elbow and gently assist. Hold for two seconds and release. Return the arm to the side after each repetition. Repeat eight to ten times. Repeat with the left arm.

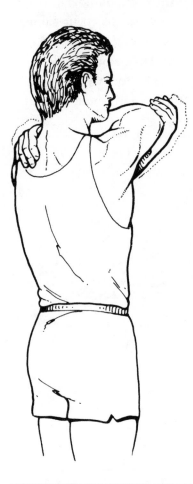

26–17. Horizontal Flexion

18. Forward Elevation

Stand and put your hands at your sides. With your elbows locked and your palms facing each other throughout the movement, rotate your right arm forward. Continue the rotation over your head and as far back as possible. Push your left arm backward in the opposite direction as far as possible. Contract the abdominal muscles to stabilize your back. Do not arch your back or allow your elbows to bend. Hold for two seconds and release. Alternate left and right arms for ten repetitions each.

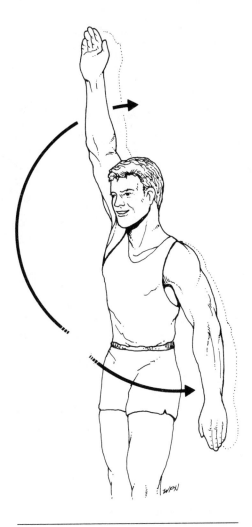

26–18. Forward Elevation

19. Triceps Stretch

In the standing position, bring your right arm forward level with your shoulder, your palm facing your body, and your elbow bent. Rotate your right arm over your head and as far back as possible. Assist by pushing your right triceps with your left hand. Hold for two seconds and release. Repeat ten times. Repeat with your left arm.

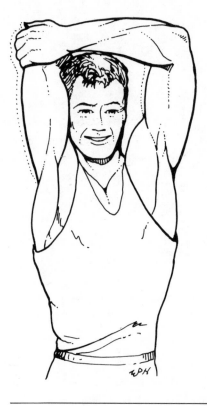

26–19. Triceps Stretch

Postscript

"ARNOLD, ARNOLD, ARNOLD," FIFTY THOUSAND SCHOOLCHILDREN screamed from the packed stands of the Baton Rouge stadium. Arnold loved it. He beamed back at the crowd from the rear deck of a convertible as it completed a victory lap around the infield. Arnold Schwarzenegger, nearing fifty, may be the primary symbol of youth in America. Arnold, more than any other living American, embodies the boundless energy, great strength, virility, and vigor that define youth. Arnold's biological clock must be permanently frozen at age nineteen. Where runners look gaunt and wizened at Arnold's age, he maintains his prime through the twin engines of youth: a large muscle mass and a high aerobic power.

I spent part of 1992 traveling with Arnold on his fifty-state campaign for youth fitness. More than anyone of their own age or any nearby generation, Arnold was the superhero of every kid we met. He transcended generations for these kids as their parents could never do and yet he was as old as some of the grade-schooler's grandparents!

I know too many men for whom fitness is sacrifice, a laborious obligation carried out to hold off Father Time. What Arnold has taught us is that the physical life is an endless celebration of youth itself. I wrote this book not as a series prescriptions for change but as a celebration of youth. Undertaking the changes in this book, for me, has been an invigorating, adrenaline-rushing adventure. I hope that as you make this book part of your life, you'll leave behind the notion of fitness as punishment and consume each chapter with an enthusiasm that will infect your friends, family, and co-workers.

One evening at his home in Los Angeles, I asked Arnold what had transformed him into the world's number one box office star. He answered simply, "I always had a dream." As a scrawny youth, he dreamed of becoming the best bodybuilder in the world, and became Mr. Olympia seven times. He dreamed of moving to America, becoming a millionaire, a movie star, perhaps even a leading politician. Each time, he invented the dream out of thin air. The dreams drove him from one goal to the next. A great disadvantage many of us have growing up in America from birth is that we've forgotten how to dream. We're checked by standardized tests, admissions committees, guidance counselors; impressions of who we are loaded onto us like a lead-filled knapsack by teachers, bosses, and classmates. We become limited, boxed in, defined by others. You can bet that Bill Gates in high school could easily have allowed himself to be defined by classmates and teachers as a nerd or a geek. The power of his own dream transcended who others would have him be as he became the richest man in America. I hope you will create a dream for yourself and your family. I hope part of that dream sees you as stuck at twenty-one, not in the immaturity of the Peter Pan syndrome, but in your vitality and enthusiasm for life.

Back in the 1950s there was a motto: "Die young, die hard, and be the prettiest body in the cemetery." Now, in the 1990s, there is a far more telling motto: "Die young as old as you possibly can." If you're like many readers, you're between thirty and sixty. By turning back the clock you will become younger and remain younger for the rest of your life. The importance of that investment will become increasingly apparent as you enter your sixties, seventies, and eighties. You are members of only the second generation in history to live into old, old age. Long-standing youth prevents the frailty that can finally ruin those precious added years of life.

I hope you will have fun with this book. Multicultural eating is a mind- and body-transforming food adventure. Becoming a highly skilled athlete is as intoxicating as ripping a Ferrari through the gears at Monte Carlo. Buying the hottest new sports toys from rollerblades to fully suspended mountain bikes allows you to play again like a child. You should feel a new sense of awe as your fat melts away and springy young muscle sprouts. The frantic stresses of life should part in your wake as you become a stress bull, unfazed by situations mere mortals see as desperate. For all of us the clock is ticking. Now is the time to turn back the clock to become the best you've ever been.

Index

Neosource Colgan Institute Meal
Replacement Protein Shake
(Neogen), 132
New Advanced Mass Fuel (Twin
Labs), 138
New England Journal of Medicine, 179,
194
New Ultra Fuel (Twin Labs), 126
New York Mets, 189
Nitro Fuel (Twin Labs), 115, 119,
131
Nitro Fuel Ion Exchange Whey Pro-
tein Powder (Twin Labs), 138
Noll Physiological Research Center,
Pennsylvania State University,
45, 189, 303
Nonsteroidal anti-inflammatory
drugs, 190–192
Nordic skating: dynamic balance in,
288
getting good fast with, 292–297
Nordic skiing, 7, 260, 267, 271, 286
learning cues for, 293–294
marks for, 162
removal of physical impediments,
296–297. *See also* Nordic skating
Northern Italians: food of, 69
NSAIDs. *See* Nonsteroidal anti-
inflammatory drugs
Nutrition, 4, 6, 9, 11, 20, 232. *See
also* Food
Nutrition Action Healthletter, 86, 110

Oakley sports sunglasses, 186
Ohio State University, Department
of Health, Physical Education
and Recreation, 118
Okinawa, 67
Old Dominion University, 135

Older athletes, 182
and sleep, 198–204
slower recovery, 146, 188–192
speeding recovery, 192–198
training for, 195–197
Oldways Preservation and Exchange
Trust, 68
Olin skis, 222
Olive oil, 68
Onboard feedback, 228–229, 244,
294
O'Neil, Bob, 339
Opti Fuel 2, 41, 114, 118
Optimum Sports Nutrition (Colgan), 43
Ornish, Dr. Dean, 12, 40, 63
Eat More, Weigh Less, 60
Otis Guy custom bike, 270
Outer calf (gastrocnemius), 377, 378
Overend, Ned, 276, 279, 280, 282
Overhead press, 316, 321
Overhead triceps press, 335, 336
Overtraining, 135, 146, 173, 174, 195

Paffenbarger, Dr. Ralph, 305–306
Palmer, Arnold, 16
Parallel dip, 321, 324
Parrillo, John, 85, 127
Parrillo (Parrillo Performance), 127
Parrillo Bars, 40
Parrillo Hi Protein Powder (Parrillo),
139
Pastas, 31, 36, 43, 63, 92
Paul Marchese, 254
Pavelka, Ed, 278, 284
Pectorals, 306, 318, 324, 325
Pelvic Tilt I and II, 366, 367
Pennsylvania State University, 118,
245
Performer (S Ski), 218
Periodization, 195, 196, 316, 350